Passionate Medicine

of related interest

Health, the Individual, and Integrated Medicine
Revisiting an Aesthetic of Health Care
David Aldridge
ISBN 1 84310 232 3

Complementary Therapies in Context
The Psychology of Healing
Helen Graham
ISBN 1 85302 640 9

Spirituality in Health Care Contexts
Edited by Helen Orchard
Foreword by Julia Neuberger
ISBN 1 85302 969 6

Spirituality, Healing and Medicine
Return to the silence
David Aldridge
ISBN 1 85302 554 2

Passionate Medicine

Making the Transition from Conventional Medicine to Homeopathy

Edited by Robin Shohet

Jessica Kingsley Publishers
London and Philadelphia

First published in 2005
by Jessica Kingsley Publishers
116 Pentonville Road
London N1 9JB, UK
and
400 Market Street, Suite 400
Philadelphia, PA 19106, USA

www.jkp.com

Library of Congress Cataloging in Publication Data
Passionate medicine : making the transition from conventional medicine to homeopathy
/ edited by Robin Shohet.
   p. cm.
   Includes bibliographic references.
   ISBN-13: 978-1-84310-298-4 (pbk.)
   ISBN-10: 1-84310-298-6 (pbk.)
   1. Homeopathic physicians--Biography. 2. Physicians--Biography. I. Shohet, Robin.
   RX61.P37 2005
   615.5'32'0922--dc22

2005006223

British Library Cataloguing in Publication Data
A CIP catalogue record for this book is available from the British Library

ISBN-13: 978 1 84310 298 4
ISBN-10: 1 84310 298 6

Printed and Bound in Great Britain by
Athenaeum Press, Gateshead, Tyne and Wear

Contents

ACKNOWLEDGEMENTS   6

Introduction   7

Introduction to Chapter 1   13
1   Following My Heart   15
Brian Kaplan, Provocative Therapy practitioner

Introduction to Chapter 2   39
2   The Medicine of Experience   41
Alice Greene, holistic medical practitioner

Introduction to Chapter 3   81
3   Medicine – A Suitable Case for Treatment?   83
David Owen, homeopathic practitioner

Introduction to Chapter 4   101
4   Seeking the True Nature   103
Peter Gregory, homeopathic veterinarian and teacher

Introduction to Chapter 5   123
5   The Betrayal of Nature   125
John Saxton, homeopathic teacher and writer

Introduction to Chapter 6   145
6   Discovering the Art of Healing – A Doctor's
    Journey   147
David Curtin, member of the faculty of homeopathy

Introduction to Chapter 7   165
7   My Journey into Medicine   167
Charles Forsyth, holistic practitioner

CONTRIBUTORS   187

THE HOMEOPATHIC PROFESSIONALS
TEACHING GROUP (HPTG)   191

Acknowledgements

First and foremost I would like to acknowledge the seven members of the Homeopathic Professionals Teaching Group (HPTG) with whom I worked for five years and whose work inspired me to edit this book. As well as friendship, we have shared similar approaches to healing which include a spiritual dimension.

Second to my partner Joan for her continued support and feedback. I have always trusted her judgment and appreciated her directness.

Third to my colleagues Peter Hawkins and Judy Ryde for their friendship and for offering their home as a retreat to enable us to finish the book.

And finally Sheila Ryan, whose comment that HPTG were pioneers helped me to decide to collect their stories.

Introduction

Collected in this book are the life stories of five doctors and two veterinary surgeons. Their search for more effective ways of healing has led them on journeys which have taken them well beyond their conventional medical training. Most of their stories are intensely personal, and yet they have a universal quality. For questions of health, sickness and cure are relevant to us all. In describing their journeys and their passions, the authors are willing to share some of their uncertainties along the way in a manner that I have found to be inspiring. It releases them (and us as readers) from the tyranny of a need for certainty which can stop us admitting to mistakes and learning from them. From knowing the authors and reading their stories, I believe that their patients and the students they have taught have benefited from their honesty and their commitment to continue learning together.

Ingrained in many of us is the idea that to be effective we have to be detached, clinical, objective; that we should not bring the feeling, intuitive side of ourselves into the consulting room and we should not recognise how the physician–patient relationship plays an important part in the healing process. Modern physics is now showing that this is an impossiblity, and that all life is interconnected so that we cannot detach the observer from the observed. However, the belief lingers on that if we take ourselves and our feelings out of the equation, we can do our job better. The authors demonstrate the cost to them, and perhaps the medical profession as a whole, of this belief.

The five doctors and the two veterinary surgeons are members of an organisation called the Homeopathic Professionals Teaching Group (HPTG, previously known as the Homeopathic Physicians Teaching Group). When the organisation was formed in 1992 its aim was to train doctors in homeopathy and a few years later this was extended to veterinary surgeons. What makes their journeys so remarkable is not simply that they have chosen to teach homeopathy in a very thorough and new way, offering courses at many different levels, or that they were pioneers in doing this for doctors and veterinary surgeons. What has moved me to collect their stories is, first, their willingness to understand the importance of relationship as a central part of the healing process. (One of the authors, Brian Kaplan, has made this the theme of his book, *The Homeopathic Conversation*.) This means that they need to be very present for every consultation. And second, their adoption of an approach which goes beyond the treatment of symptoms and aims to see their patients' potential for self-healing. To do this they have had to have a strong desire to keep learning themselves, and not allow the heavy demands put on them to make them go stale, or go into some sort of automatic pilot where they could be in danger of burn-out.

In the introduction to a book called *The Courage to Teach* (1998), Parker Palmer writes:

> Teaching, like any human activity, emerges from one's inwardness, for better or worse... Viewed from this angle, it holds a mirror to the soul. If I am willing to look in that mirror, and not run from what I see, I have a chance to gain self knowledge – *and knowing myself is as crucial to good teaching as knowing my students and my subject.* [Italics added]

I believe this applies to all those in the helping professions. From the beginning the founder members of HPTG realised that if they did not continue to work on the relationships with themselves and each other, the quality of the face-to-face work with patients would suffer, and their teaching would not develop. Through their openness to ongoing learning, they kept their passions alive and developed new knowledge and insights to increase their effectiveness. They recognised in Palmer's words the value of inwardness and knowing oneself as part of the healing relationship.

I was invited to work with them in 1999 when I received a request to be their group supervisor. This involved their bringing dilemmas in their work and their teaching to the group, situations where they felt they might not be working to the best of their ability. In this forum of frank and open sharing, new ideas could be put forward with the overall aim of going back to their work with a fresh approach. Very often this would involve looking into the mirror of self-reflection to understand where and why they might be stuck, as well as sharing their knowledge of homeopathy. It was not always easy to be vulnerable in presenting their work to others, especially when it was not going as well as they would have wished, and I admired their commitment to making regular supervision a vital part of their work.

I am passionate about the value of supervision. It gives me and the supervisee(s) the opportunity to develop a relationship which can re-engage them with the delight and joy that brought them into their work in the first place. I was lucky enough to start my professional life as a residential social worker in a team where supervision was built into the work. We were very enthusiastic about the value of ongoing learning and meeting to share our feelings about the work if we felt that it would help us to understand our client group better. Through this sharing and support we avoided burn-out from this demanding work.

My extensive experience of work with those in the helping professions – be they teachers, probation officers, nurses, youth workers, occupational therapists or doctors – is that it is rarely the work with patients alone that contributes to burn-out, but our relationships with colleagues and ultimately with ourselves. And so, as a supervisor, I not only help with client work, but also encourage people to examine some of their core beliefs which may not be serving them. Some of these might include: 'I have to know all the answers' or 'I must always be strong' or 'Vulnerability is a sign of weakness'. These ingrained, irrational beliefs can be very demanding of us and those we are close to, and take up a lot of our energy. To bring them out into the open and show how they are affecting us is often a great relief.

The authors have been very committed to this approach of working on themselves and their relationships. This has clearly contributed to the integrity of their work. It shows in their willingness to tell their stories and talk openly about what is important to them. There are common threads in many of the stories: an unhappiness with the way they had been taught, which seemed to promote insensitivity and overemphasise control and interference in the innate healing powers of humans and animals; their excitement at discovering an alternative way of treating with homeopathy and being able to work in a holistic way; their spiritual seeking; and their wish, as pioneers, to share their learning with others.

The chances are that most of us will go for treatment for an ailment some time in our lives. I would personally prefer to go to someone who has had the benefit of a conventional training, but who also has a passion for new learning that has taken them further. Someone who is constantly willing to learn and is aware of their own shortcomings, so that their patients and students are not affected by any of the blind spots that we all inevitably have as human beings.

You can enjoy these stories for themselves, but you may also wish to reflect on the ways in which they might be relevant to your own life – whether as doctor, vet, patient, student or teacher of medicine or homeopathy, or simply a seeker for new ways of healing.

References

Kaplan, B. (2001) *The Homeopathic Conversation: The Art of Taking the Case.* London: Natural Medicine Press.

Palmer, P.J. (1998) *The Courage to Teach: Exploring the Inner Landscape of a Teacher's Life.* San Fransisco: Jossey-Bass.

Introduction to Chapter 1

Brian's journey takes him from the disillusionment of medical school, discovering homeopathy and leaving South Africa, to finding like-minded colleagues and finally to Provocative Therapy, which he sees as a way of encouraging the self-healing capacity of patients through laughter.

I asked Brian what was the most important message he would like the reader to take away from his writing and he replied:

> Whether they are aware of it or not, we human beings are constantly presented with a choice of whether to follow our hearts or our heads. The wise often counsel us to pay attention to both. Orthodox medicine, based upon mechanistic science, is very much a 'head game' but once you start talking to patients, the heart inevitably enters the picture. Some doctors 'detach' and cut themselves off from their feelings in order to get through the day without burning out. I would rather find another profession than succumb to this.
>
> If there is one thing that I have learned about being a doctor and being a member of the Homeopathic Professionals Teaching Group (HPTG) it is this: when I enter my consulting room I do not walk in as a medically educated product. I am there as a human being who is prepared to make available to my patient anything I have learned in my short time on the planet, not only what they taught me in medical school. Such an attitude is equally applicable in all professions and vocations. I recommend it.

Chapter 1

Following My Heart
Brian Kaplan

'Black with milk, please,' said Uncle Louis, our beloved family GP. He had just accepted my mother's offer of a cup of tea and had been asked whether he wanted it 'black or white'. It was a typical comment from a warm-hearted man whose affection for our family was obvious. He had brought my mother, my two sisters and me into the world – so he knew us pretty well. We were made to feel special, but living in the small seaside town in which I grew up there were many others who were also made to feel special. After a while it started to dawn on me that it was he, Uncle Louis, who was special: a special doctor.

But what was so special about him? I guess he had average clinical ability as a physician. No special qualifications, although he did personally deliver a lot of babies. I believe he really loved being a GP, loved being a doctor, loved being able to be of service, just loved. And we were just another family who loved him back. Eventually our lives diverged and we left town, but I was very proud of the letter of recommendation he wrote for me when I applied to become a medical student.

So I grew up with only one idea of a doctor: a smiling, gentle, helpful and effective man who loved his work. Looking back I can now see that he was the only person I knew who loved his work so much. It was this enthusiasm for the job and the love of his patients that made me want to become a doctor.

Getting into medical school was the easy part. I just had to achieve good grades at school, which wasn't difficult. When I arrived, I learned that the reality of becoming a doctor was very different from my fantasy. I wonder how many other students have had similar experiences. I'd followed my heart but not my head and when you do that you don't always arrive where you expect! If I'd given it any thought, I would have realised that it was totally unrealistic to be expected to be taught how to be a good doctor by a bunch of Uncle Louis's! And I certainly wasn't!

I was fortunate enough to be accepted into one of the two best medical schools in South Africa. However, my elation soon ended after one year on campus. As soon as we started learning anatomy (by having to dissect a cadaver), I began to lose enthusiasm for the whole experience. I now see it as an important part of my education but at the time, dissection seemed a million miles away from the reason I had become a medical student. Committing long, complicated cycles of physiological chemistry to memory was even worse. I simply did not understand the necessity for all this detailed study of cells, tissues and organs. Five years of the six-year programme were awful for me because I couldn't articulate why I was so unhappy. After all, I was pursuing my dream of becoming a doctor, wasn't I? So why was I so miserable? Miserable or not, I still managed to pass every exam without ever having to re-sit one. This was no mean feat considering that I found the material somewhat less than inspiring.

It would take me a decade or two to realise that I was unhappy because I'd entered into the arena of medical science where patients were effectively treated as objects of science. We were advised to avoid doing this but were taught little but science. That was the problem for me. Had there been some talk of how we were feeling about becoming doctors, how we felt about medical school and all its travails or how we felt about death and disease, things might have been different. Nobody seemed to care about how I felt about anything. Why should they? They had their own careers to nurture. An honest registrar confided to me how things worked in the major teaching hospital at which I was attending ward rounds: 'Everyone here licks the arse of the person above them and kicks the backside of the person below them!' What a place to learn to become a healer! But where else was I to go?

After six gruelling academic years, I finally qualified as a medical doctor. Ahead of me lay the famous house or intern year. These were the bad old days when junior doctors did 110-hour weeks with shifts sometimes lasting 36 hours or more. Strangely enough, things started to feel better. I suppose I had a little independence and could say what I liked to my own patients in my own time!

One ward round remains forever etched in my memory. It was the morning round after being up all night admitting patients to a very busy medical ward. The entourage of white-coated doctors arrived at the bed of a man in his mid-60s admitted for acute asthma. Connected to drips, he wheezed away as his doctor presented the case to the rest of us. The patient exuded anxiety and fear. A few practical decisions were made about his medical management. Asthma is usually a mild disease but on occasion can be fatal. Treatment options for physicians are limited – so not much to think about, especially when you are practising mechanistic medicine where the mind–body connection is, at best, paid lip service. And there were 30 more cases to see before we could get started on the real work of the day. We moved down the row of beds and saw a few more cases. Then our medical registrar whispered to us: 'Don't all look at once,' she said, 'but our asthmatic gentleman has made a rather sudden improvement!' So of course everyone looked over to his bed at the same time. Amazingly, he did look a lot better, chatting away to other patients. Then he saw us looking at him and at once he started to huff and puff again. Everyone on the ward round laughed, but was this merely funny? In reality, I had just received my first lesson in holistic medicine. I had just seen, first-hand, the incredibly powerful effect the mind could have over the body. But why weren't we using this? It was a good question; a question that would fuel my journey towards becoming a different sort of doctor altogether. A doctor, not merely a practitioner of medical science; a doctor who related to his patients, even loved them: a doctor like Uncle Louis.

Towards the end of my year as a junior intern, all my friends seemed to be jockeying for positions in the great medical rat race. All talk was about careers and new jobs. Many planned to go abroad. I made no plans, but with growing excitement I knew the end was in sight. I could get out of the clutches of hospital medicine and look for something else. But what?

I had always been interested in yoga and one day I was browsing in a shop called Aquarius in van der Merwe Street in Johannesburg. There was a big box of books on sale, one of them called *Homoeopathy* (Gordon-Ross 1976). I'd heard of homeopathy, mainly used by medical consultants to deride an over-cautious dose of medication. 'That's a homeopathic [with sneer] dose!' What struck me about this book was that a medical doctor had written it. I had thought it was just quacks who used this stuff. It was on sale for next to nothing so I bought and read it. Written by a Dr Gordon-Ross, the book told the story of a doctor who had really enjoyed his work as a homeopathic GP. The book was very basic but what made me devour it in one reading was the sheer love this doctor had for his patients, his work and for homoeopathy. Here was a doctor practising medicine with passion!

As I got close to the end of the book, I felt excited and hopeful. A certain energy had been re-awakened in me. It was the energy that had driven me to become a doctor. Whatever this homeopathy was, it resonated with me in a way nothing had in seven years of medical training. At the end of the book, which I'd read in semi-trance in one sitting over a few hours, the author invited any young doctor interested in learning more about homeopathy to write to the Faculty of Homeo-pathy in London. I sent off a letter, my first letter abroad. I didn't have much: no job, no money, no career and no girl-friend. But I had hope and enthusiasm and somewhere deep inside myself, I felt blessed.

London was a revelation to me and I'm not talking about medicine. First of all, it was wonderful to live in a country that was relatively free instead of one run by a fearful, paranoid and racist minority government. London seduced me immediately as a wondrous, cosmopolitan city, a magical blend of every-thing good in the world. Naïve perhaps, but for a 25-year-old doctor, it's a good thing to be idealistic when starting out in life; cynicism can be reserved for one's later years…

It was the glorious summer of 1982 and when the sun shines, England becomes a truly magnificent country. This is because most of the time a ceiling of dark clouds closes everyone in on this small island. When the skies are blue, infinity becomes available, flowers and pretty girls appear everywhere. People smile a lot more and say, 'Isn't it a nice day?' In South Africa and California, where such days are the norm, you don't get this improvement of mood on a fine day.

To appreciate good weather, you need to suffer bad weather most of the time, it seems.

It wasn't only the weather that cheered me up. I loved the cultural scene, especially theatre and stand-up comedy. I went often to see theatre of a quality beyond my wildest dreams. I was so enamoured with the theatre that I got a reputation for using too many superlatives. Shakespeare came alive for me in quite a new way and I even began to feel comfortable with iambic pentameter! Lacking the English touch for under-statement, I praised everything I saw until one day, the mother in the family with whom I was lodging said: 'Brian, they are just actors doing their job. You do your job as a doctor and you may be doing something more important than they.' She had a point but I was unconvinced. There are many good doctors in the world but few excellent actors. Watch television every night and make up your own mind. My fascination with the theatre felt significant but I did not know why.

In October 1982, I made my way to the Royal London Homoeopathic Hospital in Queen's Square. It was autumn and there were beautiful brown leaves everywhere. Time to start studying homeopathy. I was soon introduced to my fellow students. There were eight of us, all doctors with an interesting path that had culminated in the beautiful wood-panelled room of the library at the hospital. We would spend the next six months together studying homeopathy. Among these doctors was David Owen, whose story you can also read in this book. Alice Greene was a registrar in the hospital, having done the same course as us a little earlier. I determined to get stuck into the subject matter and for the first time in my life I felt what a student is surely meant to feel – enthusiasm for the subject he is studying. Nobody pushed me. I studied out of pure passion and love of the subject. There was an examination waiting for me at the end of six months but I had no anxiety about that. If I could pass exams in subjects that were of peripheral interest to me, then what were the odds on me passing an exam in a subject I loved?

Homeopathy was the main focus of my study, but I was interested in all forms of holistic medicine. I learned some rudimentary acupuncture, naturopathy (including fasting), Bach flower remedies and healing and hypnosis, but homeopathy remained my first love. I really appreciated the respect that homeopathy gave to the patient's subjective experience of his illness and his life.

Conventional medicine never seemed to be interested in how a patient felt about having asthma or any other debilitating illness. It was interested only in objective information, which could lead to an objective diagnosis, which could then be treated with medicines proven to be helpful to that condition by objective scientific tests. In practice this amounted to finding the right pigeonhole in which to put the patient and then applying the medicine usually given to everyone in that pigeonhole.

Now, in many situations this is not a bad thing. If you have acute appendicitis you want it objectively diagnosed and treated with the standard treatment all appendicitis sufferers should get: surgery. The same goes for syphilis and pneumococcal meningitis, except in these conditions the treatment is penicillin. I'd spent enough time in the wards to know that there are times when orthodox medicine is capable of miraculous cures. The problem was that in everyday general practice these 'miracle cures' were only possible in a small minority of cases. The average patient was suffering from conditions that were not so easily eradicated by objective medical science. At last I was learning a new way of looking at the 'average patient' in a way that respected his or her individuality. This is not to say that good orthodox doctors do not respect their patients as individuals. They certainly do and our Uncle Louis was an excellent example of an orthodox doctor with a holistic approach, even though he did not use a holistic tool like homeopathy, which stimulates the body's self-healing capacity.

Over the years many conventional doctors had described themselves as practising holistic medicine, but without using any form of alternative or complementary medicine. And it's true; you can do this but you will be limited to a great degree by the tools at your disposal. You may have a whole-person approach as an orthodox doctor and love your patients very much, but when it comes to using the tools of your trade, you will have to become objective, diagnose an illness and recommend the appropriate treatment. In my opinion, a doctor becoming more holistic in his approach must acquire at least one holistic tool to use in practice. This could be acupuncture, naturopathy, hypnotherapy, counselling, autogenic therapy, meditation, yoga therapy or one of many others. A holistic tool can be defined as a therapeutic intervention aimed at the patient as a whole organism as well as at his or her symptoms. My choice of holistic tool was homeopathy. I loved the fact that in homeopathy the patient's subjective account of how he feels and how he got ill is the very essence of the knowledge the doctor needs in order to give an effective homeopathic prescription. Acupuncturists have the tongue and the pulses to turn to, but classical homeopaths are obliged to do their utmost to relate to their patients' life stories in order to find the remedy that fits those stories.

In order to do this I began to see a film of my patient's life story inside my head as he or she began to talk. Of course, the film in my head was different from what had actually unfolded in the patient's life, but as I practised this, I became better at it. I was able to judge how accurate I was by asking a few straightforward questions. I studied the Materia Medica (the medicines) of homeopathy every night for six months, as I knew this was the area they would test in the examination for membership of the Faculty of Homeopathy. For once I didn't have to cram the knowledge into my head in a frenetic, last-minute rush. This time I knew I would pass and in March 1983, I did.

During my time at the Royal London Homoeopathic Hospital, I had many good teachers who each had something to teach me. I learned about: whole person homeopathy, the history and philosophy of homeopathy, the central text of homeopathy (the *Organon*), the anthroposophical approach and the fascinating interplay between homeopathy and myth.

It was one consultant in particular who would change the way I saw medicine and myself forever. Dr Eric Ledermann had qualified as a doctor in 1932. The very next year, after an unpleasant encounter with the Nazis, he fled Germany for Scotland and managed the get the rest of his family out in 1939. After re-qualifying as a doctor in Edinburgh, he studied naturopathy and homeopathy intensively. Later he became a psychiatrist and when I met De Ledermann in 1982 he was Fellow of both the Royal Society of Psychiatrists and the Faculty of Homeopathy. As if all this was not enough, his primary interests in medicine were the philopsophy of science and medical ethics.

Dr Ledermann made me trawl through books on philosophy and psychology as well as many of his own publications (see www.wholepersonmedicine.co.uk for details). This was hard work indeed, but the significance of doing it was always clear to me. I thought back to my second year of medical school where we dissected a dead body six times a week and had to commit long lists of branches of arteries, veins and nerves to memory. At the time, I knew that the punishing detail would neither serve me nor be remembered. Studying the philosophy of science, with all its jargon (e.g. epistemology, teleology and phenomenology) was tough – writers like Kant and Husserl are not exactly easy reading! I was privileged however to be guided through their writings, so I didn't have to read long portions of unintelligible text.

Dr Ledermann was my first mentor as a medical doctor and was as often stern with me as he was totally generous with his time. The main point was that I'd found a teacher whom I could totally respect. It had been a long journey, but there is that old saying: 'When the pupil is ready, the teacher appears.'

At last I was pushed to ask myself what the doctor–patient relationship was all about. Dr Ledermann supervised my cases and by example showed me what stuff a good doctor should be made of. Doctors need to have a philosophy when they enter the clinic to see patients. Many doctors would disagree, stating simply that they are guided by 'common sense'. Dr Ledermann made me laugh by calling this the philosophy of 'Naïve Realism'!

In the end I found myself most comfortable with the works of the existential philosophers, particularly Karl Jaspers, who was both medical doctor and philosopher. He was also a major influence on Dr Ledermann and helped him to formulate his own existential approach to psychotherapy.

Dr Ledermann's simple existential ethic, which underpins his psychotherapeutic approach, has never left me. Stated simply, it insists that all patients have a conscience. Deep within themselves they can distinguish between right and wrong and know what they need to do with their lives. This is axiomatic and the only exceptions are psychopaths. Psychotic patients have a conscience but are obviously limited in their ability to make contact with it. The conscience of the patient is always at least partly unconscious. If it were totally conscious, the patient would know what to do and not consult a psychotherapist! The challenge for a psychotherapist is to help make the unconscious conscience of the patient, conscious. Understanding this was a revelation: the answer to a patient's problems is already within the patient.

This period had profound ramifications on my career as a doctor and homeopath. I began to realise that consultations with patients were not simply a matter of me choosing the correct homeopathic remedy. Sometimes, in consultation, I had felt as if the patient's job was to empty on to my desk, a whole lot of symptoms like a scattered jigsaw puzzle. It would then become my job to put all the pieces together, see the 'big picture' and prescribe the homeopathic remedy that fitted. An awesome responsibility for the homeopath and a chance to offload for the patient. There is nothing inherently wrong with this process except that the patient doesn't have to do much for him or herself in order to get better. After sitting in on Dr Ledermann's clinic for a year, I began to see the whole homeopath–patient relationship in a completely new light. I still felt some pressure to come up with the right remedy, but now I always asked myself two questions during each consultation: 'What can I do for this person?' and 'What can they do for themselves?' The second question is crucial and empowering for the patient. There is always something a patient can do to help him or herself: improve their diet, exercise, relax, meditate, work on relationships etc. Of course, if you have appendicitis or meningitis, surgery and antibiotics are, respectively, the usual treatments of choice, but for most people who consult a doctor, there is a something, however small, that they can do for themselves.

A decade or so later, I would find a potent way to motivate patients to do what they needed to do, but I jump ahead of myself…

After qualifying as a 'homeopathic doctor' (MFHom – Member of the Faculty of Homeopathy), I soon realised that I knew very little homeopathy! Sure, I had some theoretical knowledge, but would you allow yourself to be operated on by a surgeon who only knew the theory of a particular operation?

I decided I needed more training. As the doctor–patient relationship was always my first love in medicine, I enrolled on a course of Rogerian counselling run by a London university. It was one of the finest things I ever did for myself. Suddenly the therapist–client relationship was centre stage. Rogers' great contribution to the world of psychotherapy was this: results in therapy are less dependent on psychological theory and more on the very presence of the therapist. In particular, the therapist should endeavour to bring three qualities to the consulting room: warmth, understanding and authenticity. The problem is that you can't really act any of these – you have to *be* them. I grappled with this and found myself making a crucial decision about my career as a doctor. From then on I knew that I would not be doing my job well if I simply walked into the consulting room and made available to the patient everything I'd learned at medical school. That simply wasn't good enough. Not for me and not for my patients. No, I would have to make available everything I had learned about this thing we call life. Everything I'd learned from textbooks and everything I'd learned from living itself. Even from painful experiences; especially from painful personal experiences! It was a big decision but one which brought considerable relief to me. At last I felt as if I was heading in the right direction, in the direction of becoming myself. Or as Rogers might put it: 'on becoming a person'.

In addition to this course I also came to hear of the great classical homeopath, George Vithoulkas. Although not a doctor himself, for the best part of 20 years he had supervised a team of medical doctors studying homeopathy in Athens. His prowess as an accurate prescriber was legendary. However, what impressed me about him most was his holistic attitude to homeopathy. Much more than anyone who had taught me so far, Vithoulkas was totally focused on matching a homeopathic remedy to the whole human being. I studied intensively with him both in Athens and in London and learned a great deal. I liked the way he spoke with patients, making them feel that there was nothing more important in the world than that he should understand them fully. The five or six times that I attended seminars on the lovely Greek island of Alonissos where Vithoulkas lives will remain forever etched in my mind as inspiring and happy times. I made many friends there too and will always be grateful to him for showing me just how holistic an approach homeopathy really is.

After practising for a couple of years, I received very special recognition. One of my teachers from my time at the Royal London Homoeopathic Hospital, Dr Marianne Harling, invited me to help with a book she had been commissioned to edit. It was a collection of essays on Materia Medica by the late Dr Douglas Gibson. I spent several weekends at Marianne Harling's home, in the sleepy but beautiful seaside town of Bournemouth. It was an honour and a pleasure to work with her and the result was a successful book published in 1987 called *Studies of Homeopathic Remedies* (Gibson 1987). I was credited as co-editor and felt happy at having done something worthwhile. Homeopaths everywhere speak well of this book, but of course the real credit goes to Dr Gibson.

I continued to study homeopathy and attend seminars and I also became more motivated to learn new ways of helping patients help themselves. I learned about the importance of a healthy diet and exercise. One day a colleague of mine told me that one of my patients had consulted him and complained that I'd given her too much to do. I looked at her notes and saw that in addition to homeopathy I'd prescribed a strict diet, skin brushing and daily cold showers. And she repays all my hard work by not coming back, I thought. So I learned to see things from the patient's point of view and only prescribed regimens that I thought had a good chance of being carried out. All part of the learning process; all grist for the mill.

In 1975, as a first-year medical student, I had studied transcendental meditation (TM) and had benefited a great deal from this powerful technique. I knew that many patients were under a huge amount of stress and that dealing with that stress could only alleviate their condition. I hesitated to recommend TM as I knew that it had religious connections and was promoted by a well-known guru, Maharishi Mahesh Yogi. Although I was no disciple, I did not feel comfortable sitting in a Western medical practice and prescribing something connected to any religion.

My teacher, Dr Ledermann, had mentioned something called autogenic training (now called autogenic therapy or AT); a systematic form of very deep relaxation that had been developed by Dr Johannes Schulz in Germany. He didn't teach me how to do it but I knew that Dr Alice Greene, one of my homeopathic colleagues and a co-author of this book, was teaching a course. Alice was kind enough to accept me as a pupil on her course and I learned how to achieve a very quiet state of mind and body. I later learned how to teach AT and have used it ever since in my practice.

Statistics show that the great majority of patients consulting GPs are suffering from complaints either caused or exacerbated by stress. It remains a mystery why, in the light of this well-established evidence, doctors do not teach their patients how to manage stress. In my opinion, the waiting room of every general practice in England could be used to teach AT to patients every night of the week! Crazy? I don't think so. After all, the word 'doctor' actually means teacher. Tell patients to relax? They've heard it all before. Invite them to relaxation classes? Now they have a choice: should I do something to help myself or should I change my doctor?

One day in 1989 I received a phone call from a doctor called Lee Holland. He, like a few others including myself, had fallen under the spell of that maestro of classical homeopathy, George Vithoulkas. Holland was keen to form a group of doctors who would teach and promote a more classical, whole-person orientated homeopathy. I leapt at the chance and very soon after that the Homeopathic Physicians Teaching Group (HPTG) was formed. We were eight doctors who were itching to pass on this type of homeopathy to others and we were carried through to success on a wave of shared enthusiasm.

At the HPTG we achieved much. A decade after we had come together, British homeopathy had definitely swung towards the classical, whole-person approach and I believe we were influential in this. Lee Holland's dream was really coming true when tragically he died in an motorbike accident in 1996. We were devastated but united in the belief that he would have wanted us to carry on the good work. Another two members of the original group left and suddenly we were five.

From the start we had made a wise decision at the HPTG. We employed a group analyst to sit with us for two hours every couple of months. This helped us deal with many issues, including our changing personnel. The group continues and its honesty and authenticity makes it a part of my life that I will always value enormously. It is a simple process of dropping one's mask and being prepared to talk about one's feelings. This may not seem a lot but it's a million miles away from how doctors and other professionals normally relate to each other.

When the HPTG decided to include veterinary surgeons in their training we were delighted to welcome two veterinary teachers into the group and many vibrant discussions ensued. This helped us all become more empathic towards each other and I feel privileged to belong to an organisation that functions at this level. Every minute spent relating in this way feels right, although we also each have our moments of discomfort! When you use your sense of self in medicine, these are the clinical meetings you need to attend. In pure orthodox medicine such meetings would be dismissed, whereas an X-ray meeting where everyone looks at radiographs would seem natural and useful. This is the difference between objective and subjective medicine. Conventional medicine is scientific and essentially objective. Homeopathy demands both a subjective and objective approach. The feelings of the homeopath during the consultation often mirror the feelings of the patient and understanding this can be helpful in choosing a medicine. However, the homeopath also needs to be objective in separating himself from the patient and objectively choosing a medicine that suits his patient.

With these fascinating issues in mind we decided to work with a psychotherapy supervisor, Robin Shohet; this entailed supervision of our clinical cases as well as group work where we dealt with our feelings towards each other. The days spent with Robin were energising and enjoyable and I realised how important and sustaining this debriefing process was to me. It seemed to epitomise what was missing from my time in medical school and hospital medicine.

In 2000, I had shown Robin the plan for a book on the process of homeopathic consultation. Many books had been written about the medicines and theory of homeopathy but little on the type of conversations homeopaths have with their patients. Robin suggested writing the book as if the reader were in conversation with me, making the relationship between the reader and myself a parallel process to the relationship the homeopath has with his or her patients. This proved to be good advice since, when the book was published (*The Homeopathic Conversation*, Kaplan 2001), many people remarked on how much they had enjoyed its conversational style. I had been honest in the book about my travels through medical school and hospital medicine into homeopathy and the HPTG and it felt good to share this adventure with others on similar journeys.

I have always loved comedy. Perhaps that's why I loved Uncle Louis so much; he made me laugh. But I acquired my sense of fun from my father, a warm-hearted person who loved to make people laugh and feel better about themselves. I grew up in a household where the Marx brothers, Chaplin, the Rat Pack, Buster Keaton, Laurel and Hardy and many others were a big influence. I would love to have studied drama, but paradoxically this would have been highly unacceptable to my parents and even to myself. How would I have made a living? How many South African actors do you know who make a living? Exactly! So I didn't even consider the possibility. Drama was a recreation, not a profession – end of story.

When I came to London in 1982, I allowed myself to indulge my love of theatre and stand-up comedy. I was enthralled but thought of myself as merely a punter. One day I recognised a stand-up comedian I had admired on stage in a London teashop: the laconic Arnold Brown. We soon became friends and struck up a deal. He could visit me for free medical advice whenever he wanted and in exchange he would take the stress out of my day by making me laugh! We both thought we had a good deal and perhaps we did. We started to chat about the links between laughter and health. Laughter has been proved to reduce muscular tension, increase immunity, help the lungs get rid of old air and reduce stress. In addition it is a good form of exercise and gives you a natural high by raising your endorphins and encephalins, the 'feel good' chemicals of the body.

Together with improvisational comedian Neil Mullarkey, Arnold and I eventually formed the Academy of Laughter and Health. After rehearsing for a year we put on a review at a London fringe theatre called *Are you feeling Funny?* Explorations into health, humour and chutzpah was performed for two nights at the New End Theatre in Hampstead. I performed under the stage name of Dr FishHead and received a good review in the *Evening Standard.* I felt elated, far prouder than I had felt after passing any number of difficult exams at university. Finally, I'd summoned up enough courage to follow my gut feeling and do what felt right for me. It's important to live like this, whatever others think, but life is much easier when others approve!

My interest in laughter and health continued and I met the famous doctor/clown immortalised by Robin Williams in the film *Patch Adams.* The author Howard Jacobson attended a seminar on the subject run by Arnold and myself, and wrote about us in his excellent book *Seriously Funny* on the ways that humour has always been healthy for any society.

In April 1996, a psychologist friend sent me details of a seminar on the use of humour in psychotherapy. Attending this seminar was the turning point in my life. An American psychotherapist called Frank Farrelly was running it and the process was called Provocative Therapy. I went down to Surrey University for the course and within minutes of seeing Farrelly demonstrate Provocative Therapy, I had a tremendous sense of 'coming home'. All the different strands of my professional interests started to fit into place. It had all been a journey that was meant to arrive at that very moment; my experience of the 'nowness' of the moment was profound.

Frank was demonstrating Provocative Therapy in 20-minute sessions. Frank and his volunteer patients were laughing together as Frank's provocations got deeper and deeper. I found myself watching some of the most unusual therapy I had ever seen and yet it seemed so compelling. I volunteered to go 'on stage' in front of the assembled group and have a session. I remember it well. He just used humour and jesting to strip away all my false constructs and myths and leave me to face the truth that I was avoiding.

The next seminar day the trainees worked in pairs. My 'therapist partner' was Phil Jeremiah, a psychiatric social worker from Birmingham. We hit it off immediately, became close friends, and after extensive training from Frank, we eventually formed BIPT, the British Institute of Provocative Therapy.

Provocative Therapy blends humour and reverse psychology into a powerful psychotherapeutic process that provokes patients into asserting themselves verbally and behaviourally. Patients seeking psychotherapy or psychiatry generally fall into two categories. The first group includes those that have a specific problem that needs to be fixed, remedied or solved. Examples of these are acute psychoses, post-traumatic stress disorder, sudden bereavement, life-threatening illnesses and many others. The other group are those patients with long-term or chronic problems which may include depression, anxiety disorders, eating disorders, relationship issues etc. While self-reflection and insight are worthy aims in and of themselves, many of both these types of patients are seeking emotional and behavioural change. Provocative Therapy is a highly effective form of rapid 'result-orientated' therapy.

In difficult situations the most natural human response is to dispense advice but of course many patients do not appreciate being told what to do – unless of course the situation is a medical emergency when they have no choice. The traditional doctor's sincere and well-meant advice often fails because patients resent obeying orders or being made to feel fearful in any way. Thus the provocative therapist chooses instead to play the devil's advocate and take the side of the problem. Warmly pointing out good reasons why the patient should keep the problem provokes him or her into prescribing his or her own solution to the problem. The patient thus assumes ownership of the solution from the beginning and because of this is much more likely to enact that solution. The whole process is based on the idea that the solutions to patients' problems lies within the patients themselves, not in the therapist. The job of the provocative therapist was to get the patient to become aware of this solution, state it and enact it. I found this whole approach in tune with my teacher, Dr Ledermann's existential psychotherapy requires the psychotherapist to help the patient get into contact with his conscience, which may be largely unconscious. To me, Ledermann's unconscious conscience was the same as the solution to the patient's problems which was already within the patient but needed to be provoked into consciousness. Provocative Therapy showed me that a mixture of humour, satire and reverse psychology was an extraordinarily powerful way of doing this.

But what about homeopathy? I find working with Provocative Therapy completely compatible with using homeopathic remedies. Without knowing that I was a homeopath, Frank Farrelly told a story of a homeopathic doctor who came up to him after a seminar and said that Provocative Therapy was 'homeopathic'. The patient presents the problem and instead of offering any sort of solution the therapist warmly and humorously offers him absurd reasons why he should keep the problem and even indulge in *more* of the aberrant behaviour he wants to change. In this way the process is similar to homeopathy which uses medicines that are capable of producing the symptoms the patient already has. Did I need any more confirmation that I was in the right place at the right time? I became very enthusiastic about Provocative Therapy and was fortunate enough to have Frank Farrelly supervise my difficult cases. This was done by telephone across the Atlantic and called 'snoopervision' by Farrelly. Once again, I felt privileged to be accepted as a pupil by a great master especially in a subject that totally suited my personality.

After about five years of including Provocative Therapy within my practice, I realised that my education as a doctor started to make sense. Medical school was tough but would always be an excellent foundation on which to build, and being a medical doctor would give kudos and credibility to future plans. Homeopathy was the perfect holistic tool to study as it taught me how to listen to people's life stories and choose remedies based on the subjective experience of their symptoms and life rather than only on my own objective judgments. Fifteen years of listening to such stories helped me enormously in my training as a provocative therapist. One is only able warmly to satirise dysfunctional behavioural patterns when one is very familiar with those patterns. Talking and listening to literally thousands of people's life stories is the best way of acquiring that familiarity.

I also feel blessed to have worked with some wonderful teachers. George Vithoulkas taught me a beautiful and pure form of classical homeopathy to which I will always remain true. Eric Ledermann gave me a central existential ethic with which to practise medicine. It was important for me to recall this when using Provocative Therapy. The purpose of psychotherapy is to make the unconscious conscience of the patient conscious. Humour can strip away the false self, leaving the patient with a clearer view of his or her own conscience. This is obvious and simple and is the reason why effective therapy happens wherever one friend helps another laugh at how seriously he is taking his problems.

Finally

In February 2003 I was deeply honoured to be made a Fellow of the Faculty of Homeopathy (FFHom). I had become a member when I passed the required examination in 1983. That was nothing; I'd always thrived on 'exam nerves'. This was very different. This was a stated recognition of my work by my peers and I'd never experienced anything like it before. I'd always been the outsider, the schoolboy without 'school spirit', the medical student with 'the wrong attitude' and finally the doctor who went 'alternative'. Now a distinguished group of my peers had decided that I deserved to be heard within their innermost circle. That sense of belonging meant a lot to me.

I will always use homeopathy; I've seen it do wonderful things in the clinic and have total respect for it as a therapeutic tool. But for me it is not a philosophy in itself, but a very useful holistic medical intervention capable of stimulating the body to heal itself, as are autogenic therapy, acupuncture, nutritional medicine and Provocative Therapy. Not everyone is happy that I use Provocative Therapy. 'Keep the day job!' say some. 'But you're a good homeopath...' say others. 'Go for it!' say the friends who sense my enthusiasm. I think I owe it to myself to give it my best shot.

I will also make myself available to teach homeopathy, preferably with the people who are co-writing this book! I've made good friends in homeopathy and met many inspiring homeopaths from all over the world. I always make a point of asking them how they got into homeopathy. Each has a story, a journey different from mine, but we always share one thing in common. We have taken a leap of faith and followed where our hearts have led us.

References

Gibson, D. (1987) *Studies of Homeopathy Remedies*. Edited by M. Harling and B. Kaplan. Beaconsfield: Beaconsfield Publishers.

Gordon-Ross, A.C. (1976) *Homeopathy: An Introductory Guide*. Wellingborough: Thorsons Publishers Ltd.

Jacobson, H. (1997) *Seriously Funny. From the Ridiculous to the Sublime*. London: Penguin Books.

Kaplan, B. (2001) *The Homeopathic Conversation. The Art of Taking the Case*. London: Natural Medicine Press.

Rogers, C. (1995) *On Becoming a Person: A Therapist's View of Psychotherapy*. Boston, MA: Houghton Mifflin.

Introduction to Chapter 2

Alice Greene's chapter, as you will realise, is much longer than the others. She justified its length by her being the only woman in the group and having to listen to the men. Now it was her turn to speak. Like the other authors, Alice takes us through medical school and we realise the dedication that doctors must have. She tells us a lot about the philosophy of homeopathy and helps us to question some of the most fundamental concepts of modern medicine (as does John Saxton later in the book). The spiritual dimension of her work runs like a thread throughout her piece.

I asked Alice what was the most important message she would like the reader to take from her writing and she replied:

> That we absolutely exist in freedom and love, that we each matter, that we are lovable, and capable of loving others as our self. This realisation, at the heart of health and healing, is the open secret that patiently waits for us behind every disease. Making this connection conscious is the creative challenge illness brings, both to the one who is sick and to the one who cares.

Chapter 2

The Medicine of Experience
Alice Greene

Wake up. Open your eyes. Notice the little things.
Discover something that you hadn't planned to find.

Anon

At the age of 17, after ten years in boarding school, I entered
the 'School of Physic' at Trinity College Dublin to study
medicine. We began with the anatomy of death. Neatly laid out
in rows on the dissecting room tables were ten preserved
cadavers awaiting our first lessons in anatomy. Through the
overwhelming fumes of the formalin preservative, making eyes
smart and throat rasp, I recognised the form of an old family
friend who had donated his body to science. I had last seen him
the year before, laughing at dinner around our large family
dining room table. I recall looking in vain for the centre of a
human being when later we carefully dissected out heart and
lungs, guts and brain. It was empty.

My earliest childhood memories remain startlingly clear to
me. Life on a large farm in Ireland in the 1950s was very
exciting. The backyard was alive with hens, chickens, peacocks,
ducks, geese, cats, dogs and horses. On the farm, cattle and
sheep grazed amid fields of wheat, barley, oats, sugar beet and

peas. With amazement, I watched hens lay, cows calve, ewes lamb and sows farrow. My first taste of medicine was witnessing the several animal emergencies that often occurred – at the difficult birthing of calves and lambs, righting pregnant ewes trapped on their backs, or disentangling cattle caught up in barbed wire. Lambs who failed to thrive or whose mothers had died were wrapped in newspaper, and laid in the warming oven of the kitchen Aga until they had recovered sufficiently to be bottle-fed. Dead chickens, kittens or goslings were buried under a laurel bush behind the tractor shed. Their little crosses made with lollipop sticks and elastic bands soon fell over.

One day, out riding with my father, his horse stumbled, catching its leg in a rabbit hole. I watched the poor animal hop painfully with its broken leg hanging. My father sadly had to fetch his gun and shoot his horse. I was shocked to see this huge mound of horse that my father had loved, lying dead on its side. This was the first time I saw him cry.

I remember playing in the back walled garden aged five years when Jim, the gardener, suddenly fell to the ground, his head landing on his folded up jacket. He didn't answer when I called, so I kicked his boot to see if he was pretending. His foot swung idly back. I knew he was 'gone', though I didn't understand then what 'dead' was. The garden was deeply peaceful so I sat and waited until somebody came to find us. Later they told me Jim had gone up to heaven. I didn't know what that meant and remember looking up at the sky for a long time afterwards, in vain.

A couple of years later, while playing on the bank of a canal, I accidently fell in. Unable to swim, I saw the navy ribbons on my pigtails swirling above me as I sank into the dark depths. My next memory is of feeling light and of being totally enfolded in love, without any fear. Moreover, I was able to breathe easily in a body that felt even closer than my physical one. After some time, my sister, also unable to swim, managed to catch hold of a plait and pull me up, by holding arms with our cousin on the bank. This simple experience took away my fear of death. It was coming back into the physical body that was uncomfortable and frightening.

So life and death mingled on the farm. People and animals just seemed to appear and disappear again in some mysterious way. The depth and richness of my early life raised lots of questions in me about who we were and what it all meant. Concern for sick animals and people developed an early sensitivity in me for suffering in any form. Both parents had trained in medicine and served as doctors in India during World War II – my father as a colonel with the Indian Medical Service and my mother as a captain with the Royal Army Medical Corps. When the war had ended, and after some years in general practice in Ireland, they inherited some land and successfully took up farming and country life. Their generous humanity enlarged by medical experience made me decide that, despite my love of arts and language, medicine was the only thing worth studying and might somehow bring me a deeper understanding of life.

My first year in medical school turned out to be a tortuous test in chemistry, physics and statistics – a world away from my simple notions of what a doctor needed to know. Feeling uninspired, I dismally failed the end of year physics exam, and thought again about reading English literature. Determined to carry on, I successfully re-sat the year and decided to continue with another five years of medical training, looking forward to the more human side of medicine.

I felt very privileged to be at medical school and I admired the medical curriculum – beginning with our study of the natural sciences and leading up to the clinical concerns of human medicine. On the whole, we were well taught.

However, it seemed to me that various subjects were just added on to each other by tradition and usage, with nobody designing the course based on the skills, knowledge and attitudes doctors would need in practice and then assessing what was needed to get us there. It all seemed a bit 'hit and miss'. I sat seemingly endless examinations along the way, churning out regurgitated facts in different disciplines like anatomy, biochemistry, physiology, genetics, pharmacology, microbiology, pathology and forensic medicine, immunology, medicine, surgery, psychiatry, obstetrics, gynaecology and paediatrics. None of these 'worlds' seemed to fit as neatly together as I had romantically imagined. There appeared little inter-departmental communication and, between lectures, we were left to find our own bewildered way through a succession of outpatient departments. The process of medical education often felt fractured and meaningless and a few students lost their way and gave up.

The mind-obliterating medical student parties were notorious for the level of alcohol and tobacco consumed – beer would literally flow down the stairs. The first lectures of the day would begin in the heavy silence of hangover. Between studies, to remain balanced, I read voraciously, wrote lots of not very good poetry and took up stone carving. Using tungsten-tipped chisels bought from the local stonemason, I carved my way through exam stress in sand and limestone, marble and alabaster. I particularly enjoyed carving chestnut and applewood, once being awarded a prize for students' sculpture at a university exhibition of art in contemporary medicine.

As our medical studies became more clinically based, matching theory and reality was a painful learning experience. Death was sanitised and turned into statistics in the post-mortem room. I remember one afternoon talking on the wards to a young 24-year-old girl with beautiful long blonde hair. She had end-stage renal failure. Two days later, when attending my first post-mortem examination, I was deeply shocked to watch the technician pull back her hair and, using an electric saw, cut through the skull to remove her brain for examination. As her facial features sagged, I remember the hairs standing up on the back of my neck in horror with the sense that I too was just a skeleton in a rubber mask. Through these and similar experiences, I felt that I became disembodied and emotionally deadened in order to survive, losing touch with something precious within me. I entered a world of science, facts and figures where we were taught little about the art of caring or healing.

Amongst the many undergraduate studies, part of our student social medicine programme involved visiting an institution for severely retarded adults. In stone-carved letters above the door, I read with some shock, 'Home for Idiots, Cretins and Imbeciles' – words imprinted on my mind to this day. We were taken down to a fluorescent-lit basement where the most severely brain-damaged were incarcerated. In the end cell of the corridor crouched a 19-year-old youth, naked but for a pair of cotton shorts, continually banging his head against the padded wall, uttering gutteral sounds. His hands were bound in cloth to prevent him gnawing his own knuckles. I saw innocence trapped in a tortured frame and couldn't help thinking that a more natural existence might have allayed some of his obvious distress. Deep questions were raised in me about such human beings, hidden from common knowledge and view. Not that I had any answers, but that my comfortable, middle-class image of man was being shattered, leaving troubled questions about the purpose of human life. Such experiences were never discussed with us.

One day, while browsing through a second-hand bookshop, I chanced upon the writings of G.I. Gurdjieff (1870–1949), the revolutionary Russian sage who saw clearly the direction in which modern civilization was heading. I was so intoxicated by what I was reading that a whole afternoon's lectures went by the board. His words touched something deep within me:

> If a man could understand all the horror of the lives of ordinary people who are turning round in a circle of insignificant interests and insignificant aims, he would understand that there can only be one thing that is serious for him – to escape from the general law – to be free. What can be serious for a man in prison who is condemned to death? Only one thing: How to save himself, how to escape: nothing else is serious. (Smith 1976, p.2)

My passion to understand more about the nature of life and death, and the possibility of human transformation led me to join a school of philosophy which initially incorporated some of Gurdjieff's ideas. The teaching – a system of meditation, knowledge and practice for self-realisation – was based on the non-dualistic philosophy of advaita vedanta (from 'a' = not, 'dvaita' = two, and 'vedanta' = culmination of knowledge), founded 1200 years ago by Adi Shankara.

I soon learnt to meditate – one of the most life affirming choices I have ever made – allowing the mind regularly to come to rest in a profound inner silence beyond words. The word meditation, from the Latin 'meditari', to contemplate, is derived from a prior Sanskrit root 'madh' meaning wisdom. I subsequently learnt that meditation is one of the most extensively researched healthy behaviours. Over 400 published papers show that the effects on body and mind move spontaneously towards healthy values, measurable not only in physiological, but also psychological terms. One notable piece of research in 1987 by a health insurance company looked specifically at meditation and medical care. The outstanding findings of this paper included 87.3 per cent less heart disease, 87.3 per cent less nervous system disease, 55.4 per cent fewer tumours, 30.4 per cent fewer infectious diseases, with 50 per cent fewer medical consultation rates in the 2000 regular meditators, when compared with 600,000 people in the insurance company's normative database over a five-year period. This study led some insurance companies in the United States, Italy and Germany to offer discounts to people who could prove they were continuing to meditate.

Memories of my seventh year as a medical student, revising for the final exams in medicine, surgery, obstetrics and gynaecology, persist like an other-worldly experience. Rising at 4.30am, I would meditate, study for ten hours a day, meditate and sleep, living on bread and cheese, yoghurt and fruit, with gallons of lemon balm tea. Towards the end, my mind became like a highly polished mirror, absorbing whole pages of text in a sort of photographic trance – a feat never since attained. I wept when I saw my name listed on the notice board after the exams. A passing professor patted me on the shoulder in commiseration. 'But I passed, I passed', I sobbed at him, still in happy shock.

At the age of 24, my life as a medical doctor began on the wards of Sir Patrick Dun's Hospital, Dublin, where both my father and mother had started many years before. The nightmare began during my first night on duty when the surgical registrar left instruction that if a certain patient survived the night, they might consider operating on him next day. I sat up all night by his bed, transfusing ten pints of blood, which bled out of him almost as fast. Despite my encourage-ment, he died at dawn. At 8.00am I went for breakfast and cried all over my toast and tea. The incident was never discussed.

I was terrified at the prospect of being medically responsible for life and death on my first night of emergency duty, but my father gently teased me out of omnipotence by telling me, 'People are either going to live or die. If going to live, they are going to live despite you. If going to die, they are going to die despite you. You just help them do either gracefully.' This thankfully put things into a more manageable perspective.

The following years were an agony of learning, anxiety, stress and exhaustion. My enduring memories of obstetrics were of wearing a rubber apron and white wellington boots for six months of bleary-eyed night duty – made tolerable by mugs of tea and toast, and playing Scrabble in the staff room between calls. Hardly a night went by without sleep being given over to stitching episiotomy wounds, making forceps deliveries, setting up intravenous drips to induce contractions or assisting with emergency caesarian sections. The worst was delivering stillbirths or spina bifida or anencephalic babies, trying to cover their brains with surgical sheets before their mothers saw them. Such happenings were rarely, if ever, discussed. But the miracle of witnessing a birth never diminished for me; often the love was palpable. Delivering lovely, healthy pink babies more than compensated for the shouting, screams and blood of the labour ward.

My next job, as casualty officer, was for six months in the Accident and Emergency department. There, down amongst all that death and dying, illness, rape, violence, murder, drunkenness, neglect, insanity, horrific traffic accidents, fractured bones and suicide attempts, there were times I felt both inspired and disgusted by human nature. I did begin to learn however that, deeper than violence and alcohol, and behind even the most painful situations, love and its distortions were usually the core issue.

My 24-hour duty rota often meant working through most of the night, since our hospital was a main casualty centre for the city. Often, I would sleep on the crash trolley fully clothed, waiting for the next emergency, rather than waste time returning to the on-call residence a block away. I always tried to meditate twice a day and, because the ego boundaries were so worn down, would often leave my body and enter a blissful state. Such experiences brought meaningful relief to me in the relentless daily diet of human trauma, but paradoxically, made me more sensitive as well.

One day a woman came to the Emergency Room with a very disfiguring skin condition, her presence frowned upon by the ward sister, who did not consider her case to be serious. Drawn in by her obvious anguish, I heard that her GP had fobbed her off with repeat prescriptions for steroid creams, thinning her skin but not helping her rash. Apart from listening to her outpouring of grief for a long time, I felt powerless and inadequate to help, and referred her as an emergency to dermatology outpatients. Three days later, I received a parcel of six Waterford cut glass wine goblets, with an unsigned note saying, 'Thank you for listening when no one else did.' This incident demonstrated to me that not all emergencies are physical, no situation beyond help. I would sometimes see 60–100 patients in a day, then roll home to bath and bed, only to repeat the performance a day later; while my fellow casualty officer, whom I rarely met, alternated his hours with mine. After three bouts of alternate 24-hour duty, we were allowed four days off before the cycle started again. I was continually exhausted, emotionally drained and, because of the strange hours, felt socially isolated and lonely.

My next job, at the Hospital for Sick Children, was to look after the babies with spina bifida in the aptly named 'Holy Angels Ward'. I was to examine each new arrival, make an initial clinical decision, based on agreed criteria, about which were to be sent for corrective surgery and have drainage valves inserted into their ventricles. The unlucky ones were to be left to nature, nursed by a dedicated ward staff, until they died – usually within weeks or months. Every morning I would have to make my rounds and measure their little skulls, expanding with blocked cerebrospinal fluid. We fed and watered them, and kept them warm with woolly caps on their grossly swollen heads. The suffering of the few parents who visited was painful to witness. Who could blame the rest for not wanting to visit?

This was the nadir of my medical career. Like everyone else, I felt useless, angry and impotent: very close to meaningless despair. After three consecutive nights on call at the weekend, having admitted dozens of critically ill children, and spent half the night setting up intravenous drips, I would return home feeling profoundly depressed. Most traumatic of all were the cases of child abuse – little anxious children with bruises, or occasionally the scars of old cigarette burns, on their skins – rocking incessantly against the sides of their cots. 'Don't get too attached to them,' the staff sister would warn her nurses, 'because it only makes it worse when they have to leave.' The human issues of the medical staff were never discussed. On the other hand, I did get to assist the surgeon in paediatric heart operations and was astonished to see those little beating hearts exposed to the wonders of reconstructive surgery.

Entering general practice was an eye-opener. I soon discovered that all my fine knowledge, acquired at such cost, stood me in little stead when faced with the demands of patients presenting with what I privately thought were often minor illnesses. I joined the newly formed general practice vocational training scheme and came to learn, through our discussions, of the depths of human suffering that often lay behind complex presentations of unrelated symptoms. I began to see that there could be no true healing without engaging heart and mind. The contrast in my medical work between patients in a leafy suburban middle-class practice and an inner city Dublin slum was huge. Pressing social problems were often reduced to the services of a prescription pad.

I was always worried about prescribing drugs and avoided it where possible, more frightened of poisoning people. One look at the long list of side effects of many medicines in common use undermined my confidence in the prevailing system I had been taught to use. I felt that I was neither really helping people get better, nor understanding why they became ill. There had to be another way.

That was when I heard about homeopathy for the first time: a natural system of medical therapeutics that stimulated the body to heal itself. It sounded strange and exotic to me – no more poisoning the body into biological submission. So, after four years of hospital and general practice, culminating in membership of the Royal College of General Practitioners, I left Ireland for England to study full time at the Royal London Homeopathic Hospital. What immediately struck me was the care and humanity of most of the doctors I met, and the emphasis they placed on the patients' exact words in describing their own mental and physical symptoms.

We were taught a host of strange homeopathic remedies; so called because they had previously been 'proven' on healthy people, i.e. by a medically selected group of volunteers who had taken that substance over time, each recording its effects upon him or her. The group's final composite of 'proving symptoms' was then formally written up under psychological and physical subheadings, to create a unique 'symptom picture' of each remedy. Hundreds of remedies have been proved in this way. The remedy whose 'symptom picture' most closely matched the multilevel symptoms of the patient was called 'the simillimum' – the most like – indicating the appropriate one to be prescribed for that individual's condition. At once the mind–body divide was bridged and I encountered holistic medicine for the first time. This was the art of medicine as I had never learnt it, far removed from the sophisticated biological engineering of modern pharmacy and the reductionist attitude of 'one drug fits all similar diagnoses'.

The extended homeopathic case history taking gave me the opportunity to listen in depth, not just with the cold rational ears of the mind, but also with the warmer, more intuitive ears of the heart. It seemed to be just here that healing took place. The respect, empathy and acceptance that flow from this heart-centred listening provide a meeting place where doctor and patient, simillimum and disease, could bring about healing. And I discovered that this worked both ways: being healed by my patients was a revolutionary and humbling concept for me.

The word 'homeopathy' comes from the Greek 'homoeios pathein', meaning 'like suffering'. A German doctor, Samuel Hahnemann (1755–1843), was the first to found a therapeutic system based exclusively upon the homeopathic principle. A brilliant man and profound thinker, he spoke eight languages and was also a notable chemist. In 1810, the first edition of his *Organon of Medicine* was published; the sixth edition was published in 1921 and the work is now world famous (Hahnemann 1982). The idea of treating 'like with like' predates Hahnemann considerably – perhaps even as far back as the primitive practice of sympathetic magic before written records existed. Treating 'like with like' is however recorded as far back as 1000BC in China where people inhaled flakes of victims' skin to confer immunity to smallpox. The principle can be traced back to the ancient Hindus, and also through early Greek thought, appearing in the temple healings at the

Aesculepian Sanctuary at Epidauros. A similar idea was reflected in the later writings of Hippocrates who stated that like to like produces neutralization (Haehl 2001) and in the 16th century by Paracelsus, who emphasised 'vis medicatrix naturae': the healing power of nature, or the inherent ability of an organism to overcome disease and disorder and regain health (Swayne 2000). Hahnemann rediscovered the principle by chance in his now famous Cinchona bark experiment, and immortalised his findings in the homeopathic 'Law of Similars' ('Simila Similibus Curentur'): 'By the most similar, may similar things be cured' (Haehl 2001, p.67).

In homeopathy, the patient's peculiar pattern of symptoms are gleaned through an extensive history taking that covers all aspects of his personality and lifestyle. These are assessed from an entirely different, 'energetic' viewpoint. Disease is not pathology as I had been taught, but a disturbance of the patient's 'vital force'. Pathology is the result. Attention is focused on neutralising the disturbed vibration pattern by giving the 'like remedy' – the simillimum – so that, as the vital force re-establishes healthy equilibrium, the symptoms resolve themselves.

The idea of the vital force is as old as humanity: a universal belief in an animating principle in man, which leaves the body at death and is responsible for its function during life, often identified with breath. In English we say spirit, from the Latin 'spiro', 'I breathe'; 'pneuma' in Greece, 'chi' in China and 'prana' in India. By whichever path it reached him, Hahnemann adopted vitalism as the basis of homeopathy. This subject still underlies much of the debate between orthodox and complementary medicine today. Whilst we recognise the remarkable successes within mainstream medicine due to science, we can also recognise that many aspects of human suffering, because existential or metaphysical, are not accessible to scientific method and so are 'conveniently' ignored.

Central to Hahnemann's many writings, his *Organon of Medicine* emphasises that diseases are unique and individual, and that symptoms are the visible evidence of hidden dynamic causes in the patient. The outer form of the medical remedy has hidden, unseen forces within it, and so must be tested on healthy people, and the symptom picture of the proven remedy is to be matched to the picture of the patient's disease symptoms, using the smallest effective dose. This last statement continues to raise scientific controversy to this day. No one has yet been able to explain how such highly diluted potencies act, even though there are well-documented scientific trials on the successful use of such potentised remedies in the treatment of hay fever and asthma. It appears that the essential dynamic energy of the remedy is somehow liberated by the process of dilution and succussion, to act therapeutically on the same plane as the disturbed vital force itself.

Sometimes, prescribing in this way seemed to accomplish near miracles, and at other times seemed to make little appreciable difference. In frustration one day, I recall blurting to my supervisor, an eminent homeopathic consultant, that I felt I would never grasp the art of repertorising symptoms, that I was just fumbling in the dark. After listening to me in silence for a moment, he replied, 'Ah yes, my dear, but when you reach my age you learn to fumble more quickly.' His humour restored mine, though many times I veered uncomfortably between two worlds of medical thought, as though a rug were being pulled from under my feet. This made me study even harder. Surely so many fine and distinguished doctors and nurses, who had dedicated their life to homeopathy, could not be completely wrong? Working as senior registrar at the hospital, I slowly learnt to reverse my usual thought patterns, away from a pathological approach, to work with what was vital, alive and healthy in the patient. To penetrate to the centre of the case usually uncovered a hidden emotional trauma or shock to the system, often denied, unconscious or repressed, making the inner planes shut down, blocking the natural energy flow. Symptoms were the expression of a hidden inward cause.

I soon learnt of a Greek master homeopath, George Vithoulkas, teaching in London and Greece, and enrolled to attend his teaching seminars with 60 or so other students. George had been a mining engineer in South Africa where one day he had chanced upon some old homeopathic books in a bookshop. Intrigued, he bought them and took them home to study. He told me his hands were burning with excitement as he read for three days. He was astonished that such a little-known system of therapeutics existed, and decided then and there to give up engineering in order to devote his life to homeopathy. After many years of travels and study, he opened a homeopathic treatment centre at Maroussi in Athens, staffed by 26 homeopathic doctors working under his guidance. Over the years, he collected and documented approximately 150,000 homeopathic clinical cases from which many important additions to homeopathic Materia Medica were made.

When George was invited to London to teach, we would watch him, via video link from another room. After taking the patient's case history, he would join us for a discussion of the homeopathic remedy needed. This was an incredibly exciting learning experience. Soon a group of us were travelling once a year for further studies to Alonissos, a Greek island in the Sporades, where George lived with his wife. It is difficult to express the soaring spirit of those days, when we felt we were being introduced to the true healing potential of homeopathy.

George's case analyses were legendary and his skill in elucidating the deeper facts of the case always impressed me. It was like going from a 'flat earth' view to a rich, multi-dimensional experience which filled us all with incredible confidence, and gave us an expanded knowledge of the many remedies at our disposal. One case, of the very many which made a vivid impression on me, was of a 30-year-old man with disabling arthritis. He always hesitated before answering questions and even then, spoke very slowly. There was nothing very significant to point to the remedy. George asked us what we had noticed. Our several tentative replies were dismissed as superficial. He then asked whether anyone had noticed the fear in this man's eyes. No one had. He turned to the man and asked him if anything very frightening had ever happened to him. The man reacted violently, seeming to struggle with great emotion and, as if coming out of a dream, began to describe something he had forgotten many years ago. Whilst working as a lifeguard in his 20s, he had been called to a boating accident on a lake. He remembered diving down into the cold murky waters when suddenly, through the reeds, he brushed up against a face with fixed staring eyes – the body, suspended upside down, was trapped below the surface by an anchor chain. In his horror, he panicked and almost drowned. This shocking memory had lain buried beneath his outer life. He had subsequently become depressed and gradually indifferent. The homeopathic remedy prescribed was phosphoric acidum, and his arthritis cleared up within a couple of months.

George has since opened his own International Academy for Classical Homeopathy, a beautiful stone building, modelled after a Byzantine monastery and built to his own design, on the island of Alonissos. Here, students travel from all over the world to study homeopathy. George was deservedly awarded the Alternative Nobel Prize, also known as the Right

Livelihood Award, in 1996, for his lifelong dedication to the cause of homeopathy worldwide.

Meanwhile, back in England, I continued work in three successive general practices in London, becoming more confident to the point where at least 40 per cent of my patients received homeopathic prescriptions. The last NHS practice in which I worked had one of the lowest drug bills in the area and attracted many people, especially women and children, who preferred homeopathy's gentler approach. I was also teaching for the Faculty of Homeopathy and it was heartening to see so many doctors make that profound shift in their awareness as the implications of the homeopathic approach went home.

I simultaneously became interested in the concepts of health and healing in traditional Indian ayurvedic medicine (from 'ayus', life, and 'veda', knowledge of). The renowned Indian physician, Charaka, compiled one of the earliest ayurvedic texts, the *Charaka Samhita* written in Sanskrit, about 1200 years ago. This text, now translated into English, forms the basis of the many ayurvedic courses currently available in the West. Two-thirds of the treatise expounds upon the natural measures for living in health and harmony, and one-third on treating diseases with herbs and surgery – an attractive balance! I found its philosophy of health and disease, and the commonsense guidelines on diet according to body type, especially practical. In one ayurvedic text, health is beautifully summed up as, 'Balance in the energies, digestion, bodily tissues, and excretion. And peace between the soul, mind and senses' (Sharma 1999, p.173).

It was precisely that important second half that seemed to be missing in modern medicine (because it seemed to be missing in many doctors) and in me. Over the years, I had discovered that my own painful experiences, far from being unique, were shared by almost every doctor I spoke to. Given the traumatic nature of medical education, in the absence of attention directed to the emotional health of doctors, it takes a small step to understand why a large majority of medical professionals are themselves wounded healers. Unless we have engaged in some form of emotional healing, we must, like any abused person, be unconsciously focused on pathology and so become unconscious abusers of others. This we do through alienation; hearing patient's anecdotal stories as irrelevant; ignoring clues of emotional distress; making 'expert' diagnoses and so treating patients as objects of science to whom we do 'expert' things; and seeing disease and death as forces to be conquered by the surgical techniques and drugs of rational science.

Not surprisingly, this lack of recognition of the links between mental and physical health are unfortunately reflected in the psychological health profile of many doctors, with drug and alcohol abuse, marital disharmony and suicide rates at much higher levels than in the general population. As for myself, I developed a serious double pneumonia and realised, while recuperating in hospital, that transcending emotional wounds in meditation, in favour of a peace beyond, didn't seem to heal the conflict between heart and mind. I needed to face whatever was blocking my inner energies.

In my reading, I had come across the works of Carl Jung (1875–1961), a Swiss psychiatrist who developed the field of analytical psychology, following his early work with Sigmund Freud, the Viennese founder of psychoanalysis. Jung's vigorous researches into all aspects of human endeavour extended his influence into the fields of anthropology, theology and philosophy. He wrote:

> We are shaken by secret shudders and dark forebodings; but we know no way out, and very few persons indeed draw the

conclusion that this time, the issue is the long-since-forgotten soul of man. (Jung 1982, p.365)

Jung (1969) famously pointed to the wisdom of our 'collective unconcious', an innate archetypal patterning organising our world consciousness, which guides all humanity. Therapy should help bring people into contact with this deeper collective unconscious, and their own healing. Having read a little of his voluminous works and admiring his spirit, I chose to sit through three years of attentive and healing Jungian analysis for which I was very grateful. Crawling out from under the emotional rocks was painful. I talked a lot, discussed significant dreams, cried, relaxed and learnt to trust my own feelings again, without projecting my pain on to others. Ongoing meditation helped integrate my understanding, so that by the end, I felt a richer human being, and more present to myself and others in daily life.

This insight into deeper levels of being and healing raised serious questions in me. I became more disillusioned by the optimistic zeal with which drug company representatives promoted their ever 'newer', more 'potent' drugs within general practice. I also came to resent the NHS straitjacket of having to see 30 patients a day, within the allotted eight to ten minutes each. More time was needed if any case was to be more deeply examined. I knew I had to change direction.

In 1986, with a small bank loan, I opened my first private practice in Hampstead, in the sitting room of a delightful family with whom I was living at the time. One day, I was amused to see through the window a man, whom I thought to be my first patient, calmly stare at my gleaming brass plate on the wall. He then took out a comb, parted and combed his hair and walked on up the hill. But people slowly came, often to talk and share their deepest feelings, spilling out their secrets, tragedies, unhappiness and pain. As part of deepening the holistic approach, I became more interested in diet and nutrition, exercise and creativity, factors to re-balance lopsided growth. It was gratifying to witness people's lives turn around and walk with them on the road to well being. Having also studied acupuncture at the Homeopathic Hospital and used it in the pain clinic, I began to use it to treat people whose stress patterns appeared to block healing. I was also impressed at how much people's illnesses improved when they learned to relax. This made me want to find a system of stress management that people could learn for themselves.

In 1987, I studied autogenic training (AT), a very simple system of self-induced profound relaxation, which can help a wide variety of common medical conditions and psychological problems, with well-researched, positive results. The six volumes on Autogenic Therapy (AT) written by Dr W. Luthe and Dr I.H. Schultz in 1969, detailing its use in clinical medicine and psychotherapy, were published in eight languages, spreading AT to many countries around the world. Brought to the UK in 1982, AT is now used in at least four NHS hospital outpatient departments with impressive results. Apart from the usefulness of AT in many clinical conditions, many people have used it in the fields of sport, education and industry. Improvements in peak performance, creative output, intellectual work and interpersonal relationships have all been recorded: by factory workers to reduce absenteeism, by Russian and US astronauts to combat zero gravity problems, by aircraft crew to overcome stress and jet-lag, by schoolchildren to improve classroom learning skills and behaviour, by the police force and ambulance service for stress reduction and the British Olympic Rifle Team to reduce performance anxiety, to name but a few. I believe its use will grow.

I recommend AT to my patients as a great way to deal with stress and take control of their lives again. Many are able to come off antidepressants, mild anti-hypertensives, analgesics, sleeping tablets and tranquillisers, and to overcome recurrent minor infections, skin problems, low self-esteem, anxiety, or general malaise. I have taught over 40 groups in the ensuing years, as well as many individuals. I joined the education and training team of the British Autogenic Society, eventually being elected chairman in 1997 and awarded Fellowship of the Society in 2001.

Another strand in my life began in 1991, at a meeting of like-minded homeopathic doctors where I presented an overview of a successful Dutch homeopathic training school for doctors. Most of us at that meeting had studied with George Vithoulkas, using a similar approach in our different homeopathic practices. As we were working in geographical isolation and outside the usual NHS career structure, we wanted to share our experiences, and to offer our collective insights to others in a more formal way. The discussion was full of energy and enthusiasm, and from it was conceived the idea of opening our own homeopathic school in Oxford. Eight doctors initially signed up as core teachers, under the name of the Homeopathic Physicians Teaching Group (HPTG).

During the next 12 years, our homeopathic courses for doctors expanded to include nurses and vets, at undergraduate and postgraduate levels. Central to all our work was the focus we put on ourselves as a partnership. Regular meetings with a group analyst ensured that our business relationships were kept consciously integrated with our core vision. We worked hard to model these values within the student groups we taught, as a way to heal some of the fragmentation we ourselves had experienced in medical education. The pioneering spirit that spurred us on was intensely creative and exciting, and we watched ourselves, our students and our course structures grow organically, to seed new ventures.

In 1999, we began running a three-year teacher training course for ten of our homeopathic graduates – just in time – since we were invited to teach homeopathy overseas, and soon successfully established HPTG International Courses in Australia and the Republic of Ireland. We are continuing to develop teaching links abroad by invitation from other interested medical and veterinary groups. Another venture was the introduction of a psychodynamic model of homeopathic supervision to the clinical world of medical and veterinary encounters. The effect was to inspire and deepen homeopathic case taking to new levels of understanding for doctor, vet and nurse.

After starting the HPTG, I became aware of the need to consolidate the many short counselling courses I had taken over the years, since I was encountering in my own practice many people who needed more time to work through their various difficulties. I successfully applied to the Psycho-synthesis and Education Trust for a three-year diploma course in counselling and therapy. As students once again, we laughed and played a lot together on the basis that 'it is never too late to have a happy childhood'. However, as the only medical doctor in our large group, I was unprepared for the amount of negative transference projected on to me by some group members who had suffered bad experiences at the hands of their own doctors. A few of the stories I heard were so frankly appalling that, at times, I felt almost ashamed to be a doctor. Becoming more aware of aspects of my own medical conditioning helped me to share with the group something of the difficulties encountered by doctors, which was helpful for us all.

These were also magical times as I saw the changes taking place in us through honestly sharing our feelings together. Being willing to recognise and transform emotional blocks usually brought mutual understanding, and spontaneously reversed painful judgments and distorted behaviour. To me, this agreed on a psychological level with the 'Law of the Direction of Cure' exemplified by a follower of Hahnemann, Dr Constantine Hering, who observed that cure usually proceeds 'from within out, from more important to less important organs, from above downwards, and in the reverse order that symptoms first arose' (Lockie 1989, p.13). These observations made me reflect on whether there was any connection between 'suppression', e.g. drugs blocking symptoms and so pushing 'disease' to deeper levels within the organism, and the phenomenal rise in mental health problems in Western society. This added impetus to my homeopathic case taking.

Another event which deeply influenced me was when I attended, on behalf of the British Autogenic Society, the XIth World Congress of Psychiatry in Hamburg in 1999. The theme of the Congress concerned the fact that, according to World Health Organisation research, psychiatric disorders now account for five of the top ten causes of disability, and for nearly 11 per cent of the total global burden of disease. By the year 2020 AD, psychiatric and neurological conditions could increase their share of the total global burden by almost 50 per cent – a forecast viewed as accurate by 70 per cent of the UK psychiatrists polled (WHO 1998).

At the Congress, a strong feature of the many presentations concerned the direction in which psychiatry is headed: will psychiatrists become neuroscientists 'treating the brain' or psychotherapists 'helping the mind'? When we move psychiatry to the laboratory, we remove it from the life of patients. Are we moving from the age of the asylum to the age of Prozac, from being healers to being gatekeepers for antidepressants?

The theme of reducing people to objects of science to whom we 'do things' was chillingly brought home to me in a way I had not anticipated. A central feature of the Congress was a memorial exhibition commemorating approximately a quarter of a million victims of the National Socialist Euthanasia Programme operating from 1930 to 1945 in Germany. Patients were killed by their doctors: by starvation, infection with TB, injections of Luminal, or with a cocktail of morphine and scopolamine to ensure respiratory failure and death. This programme was systematically carried out against the old, unfit, incurable, misfits, genetically impaired and immigrants unable to work. At the Nuremburg Medical Trials Tribunal in 1947, of the 23 medical doctors indicted for 'crimes against humanity', the chroniclers wrote that these terrible atrocities had been so chillingly organised, with such technical bureaucracy and carried out in such a malicious and bloodthirsty way that no one could read the reports about them without feeling the deepest shame. After 140 days of legal proceedings, the testimonies of 85 witnesses and almost 1,500 documents, 16 of the doctors were found guilty. Seven were sentenced to death and were executed on June 2, 1948.

This exemplified for me, in the most horrific way, the violent consequences of losing sight of our own humanity, the almost logical end-point of a science divested of human meaning or morality. This chilling experience further confirmed for me the absolute necessity for a metaphysical worldview that put the heart back into medicine – not as a sentimental gesture, but as an enlightened appreciation of the way things naturally, and lawfully, work best. And not because they should, but because they do.

Like many other people, I have often wondered about the clouds overshadowing the world in the last century and this, of world war, Holocaust, labour camps and killing fields; through enforced starvation, systematic torture, genocide, ethnic cleansing, religious persecution and political warfare. If these were all symptoms of a disease, viewed as the enlarged expression of an individual facing an existential crisis of meaning, would the direction in which science and technology are leading us save us in the end? Or, would we realise, as the Chinese proverb says, 'If we do not change our direction, we are sure to end up in the direction in which we are headed.'

It seems as if the modern cult of scientific rationale has reduced our age-old view of the cosmos, and man's place within it, down to the evidence of our physical senses alone. Is there a deeper soul truth underlying the scientific worldview? What happens to people when terrible things are done to them?

In a fascinating paper entitled *Mystical Experience of the Labour Camps*, Mihailjo Mihajlov presents remarkable evidence from many eyewitness accounts of survivors from the Soviet prison camps in the Stalinist era, which 'explodes the very foundations on which modern science and philosophy are built' (Mihajlov 1976, p.120). All the authors writing of those experiences agree that arrest and imprisonment – the loss of freedom – have formed the most profound and significant experience in their lives. Although enduring the most extreme spiritual and physical suffering, they also paradoxically experienced a fulfilling happiness undreamed of by people outside the prison walls. Those writers, who had been through the most life threatening circumstances affecting both body and soul, unanimously affirmed that:

> Those [prisoners] who sacrificed their soul to save their body lost both; while, for those who were prepared to sacrifice their body to save their soul, some kind of strange and mysterious law eluding understanding, preserved both. (p.106)

Demonstrating that the spiritual world cannot be separated from the physical, numerous accounts by prisoners tell of miraculous guidance from the depths of their souls, an inner spiritual voice which, when followed, led to freedom, and when ignored, led to death. Mihailjov says this internal voice is not subject to any intellectual criteria or scientific study, 'since the point of departure of science is the premise of the existence of only one world, ruled over specifically by the cognition of laws independent of man' (1976, p.108), although the experiences of life in captivity pointed to quite the opposite.

Mihailjov (1976) writes that sooner or later, each of us living in the world will at some time find ourselves in 'prison', either through sickness, catastrophe, misfortune or death. He points out how we are compelled, unavoidably,

> To make a choice between submission before death or, in contradiction to everything 'real', 'objective' and 'sensible', to follow in a daring way the calling of the spiritual voice… Only through complete renunciation does a person become totally free – only then, when he no longer has anything to lose… Spiritual slavery leads to prison, spiritual freedom liberates one. For, suffering opens man's eyes to the inner spiritual world, to the mystical compass found in every man's soul (p.111).

Such prisoners realised they didn't own this force, i.e. that they didn't have the right to direct it according to their own judgment but on the contrary that everything in life – and life itself – is completely dependent upon this mysterious spiritual force. The numerous experiences they reported of this mysterious fundamental law at work indicated not only a common basis for both the spiritual and physical worlds, but also that what happens in the physical world depends on what happens in the spiritual world, and not the other way around.

In light of these and similar accounts from all over the world, it follows that an over-optimistic belief in the world of science may paradoxically separate us from knowing and having faith in the simple truth within each human being: that we absolutely exist in freedom and love, that we each matter, are lovable and capable of love. Being seduced by the scientific promise of certainty can lead to ethical compromise, dulling our hearts and minds to the sharper vision of spiritual freedom within.

More than a century before, Hahnemann voiced just such concerns over the direction in which the science of his day was headed. His legacy foreshadows the rise of a holistic medicine fundamentally different from the mono-scientific approach. The discovery of more powerful 'tools' to enforce change, by interfering with natural mechanisms, can overlook the unity and wholeness of the human being and ignore or suppress the spontaneous activity of our natural healing powers.

The great spiritual seers down the ages have reminded us again and again that the final or greatest disease is ignorance of our own true nature. When a contemporary spiritual leader of the advaita tradition was asked some years ago by a group of English doctors, 'What is the real medicine?' his reply was startling. He said that all systems of medicine – Western or Eastern, Tibetan, Egyptian, Chinese or Indian – are 'outward' systems only. They will carry people for a while, or provide some temporary relief, but as long as we remain 'in ignorance' we will inevitably be surrounded by physical, mental and emotional diseases of every kind. The real medicine brings about transformation at the inner levels of being. If we really want to make the body a temple suitable for the self to do its work then we need to wake up to the reality that underlies our very being.

Hahnemann himself equated true health with freedom. One of the greatest homeopaths after Hahnemann, Dr James Tyler Kent (1849–1916), pointed out that the freedom to experience this consciousness is hampered by illness, by symptoms, in fact. He controversially said that, 'There are no "diseases", only sick people' (Kent 1979, p.22). A patient doesn't come asking for freedom; he says he is sick because he has symptoms, whereas homeopathy says he has symptoms because he is already sick. Freedom is the final cure. Vithoulkas, in an international seminar held in Alonissos, described this freedom in terms of three levels: freedom from physical pain with a sense of vitality and well being; freedom from emotional passions and negative emotion with a sense of dynamic calm; and freedom from mental selfishness and erroneous ideas with a sense of clarity and detachment, evolving through conscious effort into the divine qualities of love and wisdom. This makes sense of a holistic model of health that places spirit at the centre, giving significance, value and meaning to life and providing opportunities for realisation of our innate human potential.

In 1999, two years after the tragic death of our HPTG colleague and friend, Lee Holland, I was invited to give a memorial lecture on the theme of *Physician Heal Thyself*, at the Royal London Homoeopathic Hospital. While looking up this reference in the writings of Luke, himself a physician, I found myself reading again, with new eyes and ears, the many accounts of healing performed by Jesus:

> Don't be afraid.
> Be clean.
> Your sins are forgiven.
> Get up and walk.
> Stretch out your hand (to the man with a withered arm).
> Don't weep (to the grieving widow).
> Young man, get up.
> Your faith has saved you. Go in peace.
> Peace, be still.
> Be comforted. Your faith has made you whole. Go in peace.

Have no fear. Have faith and you will be made whole.
Receive your sight. Your faith has saved you.

Words like peace, wholeness, forgiveness, stillness, absence of fear, faith and comfort point, for me, to the heart of true healing. They express the very qualities that seem to flow when we are in touch with our common humanity, when we are most truly and profoundly ourselves. Hahnemann himself stated that:

> All human beings naturally seek happiness. The greatest of all physical goods is health, which not all the riches in the world can pay for, and the restoration and maintenance of which is man's most important and difficult concern. (Schmidt 1993, p.294)

The vital force, Hahnemann wrote, keeps the body in harmonious balance, 'so that our in-dwelling, reason-gifted mind can freely employ this living healthy instrument for the higher purposes of our existence' (Hahneman 1982, p.33). He describes 'cure' as bringing about 'a greater degree of comfort, increased calmness and freedom of the mind, higher spirits; a kind of return to the natural state' (Hahneman 1982, p.129).

One measure of health lies in our creativity. The healthy person seeks to create rather than destroy, working positively, in harmony with himself and others. Creative self-expression is naturally linked to positive feelings of meaningful self-worth. Blocking our creative energy flow is therefore more serious because it leads to frustration, depression and despair, with negative consequences for our mental well being and physical health. Rather than suppress symptoms with drugs, it is here, in the energy field of the inner mental and emotional planes, that homeopathy can work to such good effect.

Hahnemann insisted on the importance of self-knowledge in the healing process, saying that through such self-observation:

He – the physician – will be brought to understand his own sensations, his mode of thinking and his disposition (the foundation of all true wisdom: Know thyself), and he will also be trained to be, what every physician ought to be, a good observer. (Hahneman 1982, p.91)

Not only 'a good observer', but also, as Hahnemann extolled, 'an unprejudiced observer'. Within the HPTG, in response to the needs of graduates, we set up regular postgraduate supervision groups for doctors and vets. Early on, we recognised that certain attitudes and feelings, unknowingly projected by the patient onto the doctor (transference) and by the doctor onto the patient (counter-transference), could be made conscious and explored to the benefit of both. Using the 'six eyed model' of supervision we could begin to examine the worlds of the patient, practitioner and supervisor and the interactions between them. This elegant psychodynamic model provided an insightful way to uncover the blocks and projections obscuring the centre of the case. For example, a simple question like 'Who does this patient remind you of?' to a doctor describing an emotionally charged consultation, can often yield surprising and illuminating insights! Increasing awareness of the feelings elicited in the doctor by the patient (projective identification) can help uncover the deeper emotional issues involved, and radically improve prescribing. I personally hope that the medical, nursing and veterinary professions come to see the wisdom of establishing such groups. The opportunity for peer support, personal growth and self-development could help positively to transform the burden on the caring professions as a whole.

In an original paper, 'Doctors can't help much: The search for an alternative', the authors write:

Scientific medicine is making big advances in drugs, technology and genetics, yet more and more patients use complementary therapies. Evidence based medicine dominates our discourse, yet health professionals increasingly refer to and practice complementary therapies that appear to have little scientific evidence of efficacy. (Paterson and Britten 1999, p.626)

On the other hand, medical drugs with 'proven efficacy' are not the whole answer either. Dr Alan Roses, the worldwide vice president of genetics at GlaxoSmithKline was quoted in the *Guardian* in December 2003 as saying that 'more than 90% of drugs in use only work in 30–50% of the people for whom they are prescribed'. The reason for this is thought to lie in our differing genetic make-up: not good news for the 4,000 people who die each year in the UK from drug induced ulcers (half of whom have no prior symptoms to alert them to the dangers). This is double the number of deaths from asthma. There were 20,272 adverse drug reports in 1991. The Committee on Safety of Medicines (CSM) suggested this was only 10 per cent of the most serious side effects. By 2002, the percentage of serious reports, as a total of all reports received, had risen from 55 per cent to 67 per cent, according to the Committee on Safety of Medicines' 'Report on Adverse Drug Reactions' (2002). Other researchers found that only 1 in 24,000 drug reactions is ever reported by the doctor (Maride *et al.* 1997). By 2004, another study suggested that adverse drug reactions cause more than 10,000 deaths annually in the UK (Pirmohamed *et al.* 2004).

The CSM regularly publishes a long list of 'new drugs under intense surveillance', usually more powerful drugs with stronger side effects. In 1998, researchers at the University of Toronto analysed the results of 39 international prospective studies to estimate the incidence of serious and fatal adverse drug reactions in hospital patients. They calculated, using their highest estimate of the scale of the problem, that adverse drug reaction was the fourth leading cause of death, i.e. only heart disease, cancer and strokes are more dangerous. Their lowest estimate put adverse drug reaction sixth, behind pulmonary disease and accidents (Lazarou, J.L., Pomeranz, B.H. and Corey, P.N. 1998).

These statistics are a sad reflection on the first injunction of the Hippocratic oath – 'Above all, do no harm' – an oath which, until relatively recently, was a requirement for all doctors on qualification. Perhaps it was the oath's further injunction to doctors against the induction of abortion that finally withdrew it from contemporary use.

Concern about the increasing medicalisation of society led Ivan Illich to write his famously thought provoking book, *Medical Nemesis* in 1974. He found the Western cultural belief that all suffering is avoidable to be deeply misleading, and he predicted that in trying to eliminate suffering, doctors inevitably create more. We are today witnessing a rising tide of iatrogenic disease as evidence of this.

Scientific research, at the core of orthodox medicine, by trying to find chemical and biological agents to eliminate disease, may be based on a wrong fundamental premise. The real question is, how does an organism allow a disease state to occur in the first place, and how may the natural mechanisms of mind and body be best supported to resist or overcome it? Is there another way?

Paterson and Britten (1999) found that when patients with chronic disease were interviewed, their reasons for consulting complementary therapies fell into three categories. The most common was, 'Doctors can't help much'; second, 'Doctors are hopeless'; and third, 'Although the drugs may work, their side effects are not acceptable'. The authors concluded that such patients actively seek out and appreciate holistic patient-centred care, suggesting that:

not only are the big advances of scientific medicine irrelevant to these patients but that a scientific emphasis alone may be diverting doctors away from the real needs of patients with chronic disease and leaving a vacuum...which is increasingly being filled by complementary therapies. (p.626)

In another paper, 'The physician healer: Ancient magic or modern science', Dixon *et al.* write:

Our potential skills in diagnosis...have never been so great...our credibility further enhanced by a newly won bio-mechanical understanding, effective treatments and the ability to apply evidence based medicine...but something is missing as our therapeutic role over the years has slowly diminished... (Dixon *et al.* 1999, pp.309–12)

The authors point out that, 'The art of healing and the strength of the patient–doctor relationship play a vital role in the well being of the patient.' In view of this, some people suggest that homeopathy may work simply through the 'placebo response' but this is not a satisfactory answer (Reilly *et al.* 1994). While this is to some extent true of all medical encounters, it does not explain the many documented healing responses in animals when given homeopathic remedies, e.g. in kennel cough in dogs, mastitis in cows, spontaneous abortion in sows, and pneumonia in calves. Based on a European survey showing the rising use of homeopathy for pet and farm animals across Europe (because the non-toxic remedies help reduce antibiotic and other drug residues in agricultural products and animal waste), EU regulations since 1999 have recommended the use of homeopathic and plant-based medicines as the treatment of first choice in the health care of animals being raised organically (Viksveen 2003, p.104). Another study from Norway showed that 37 per cent of all farmers had used homeopathy to treat their animal herds (Viksveen 2003, p.104).

But the best research evidence for the clinical efficacy of homeopathy comes from meta-analyses, combining many human studies, to show effects at a level of certainty beyond the scope of any single study to demonstrate. Out of a number of such studies, one by Linde *et al.* (1997) analysed a total of 89 clinical trials, covering nearly 11,000 homeopathic patients. It concluded that the clinical effects of homeopathy were more than placebo effect.

Homeopathy is now widely practised across Europe. A recent survey showed it to be among the three most frequently used complementary therapies in 11 out of 14 countries, and the most frequently used in five countries. Up to a quarter of EU citizens use it, the number in France rising from 16 per cent to 36 per cent within ten years – a pattern also seen in Belgium, the Netherlands, Norway and Switzerland – mainly because of concern about conventional drug toxicity (Viksveen 2003, p.102).

Although some people argue that the case for mind–body medicine, meditation and a holistic view of health is intuitive and unscientific, there already exists a large body of scientific evidence to support it. And while 25 years ago there were only two or three academic institutions carrying out research into homeopathy, today over 100 universities and other institutions throughout the world are actively investigating homeopathy and 'low dose effects'.

Dixon *et al.* (1999) continue:

> Yet it seems the physician healer is now poised to rise again like the Phoenix, not on a wave of nostalgia, but because modern science demands it. Placebo research and psycho-neuro-immunology are beginning to clarify a role in which caring is no longer an act of compassion or indulgence, but has everything to do with curing or, in the modern term, effectiveness... The modern GP therefore needs to develop

skills as a physician healer in order to bridge the gap left by his medical science. (p.311)

The authors conclude, 'The Physician Healer is not an anachronism but a modern necessity'.

The growing popularity of homeopathy today around the world attests to this need. I am thankful to have studied both medicine and homeopathy and grateful to all my teachers, patients, colleagues and students who continue to light the way. Like all doctors, I certainly appreciate all the amazing resources of modern medical technology and appropriate life saving drugs at our disposal. Yet despite this, as Rene Dubos wrote in *So Human an Animal* over 30 years ago, many agree that 'The age of affluence, technological marvels and medical miracles is, paradoxically, the age of chronic ailments, of anxiety and even despair' (Dubos 1999, p.14).

While for me homeopathy is not the only answer, and certainly not the final answer, Hahnemann's 'medicine of experience' (Hahnemann 1982, p.xi) does provide a growing body of medical thought closer to the natural order. For me, homeopathy seems to act as a bridge between the worlds of science and healing, matter and spirit. Within its sphere, the time-bound linear logic of the left brain (oneself in the world) and the meaningful holistic imagery of the right brain (world in oneself) are reconciled. The narrative-based remedies of homeopathy, because 'proved' in ordinary human experience, can help reconnect the broken narrative threads of people's lives, to restore natural balance and promote true healing by the gradual liberation of the vital force. As John Launer writes:

> In many ways, therefore, narrative-based medicine turns the conventional biomedical approach – and even the patient-centred one – on its head. Instead of listening to 'the patient's history' to determine what to do, it judges our actions by whether they contribute to an improvement in the

patient's narrative. Philosophically, this is indeed a giant leap. (Launer 2003, p.92)

I can personally attest to the importance of this. From qualifying as a doctor full of youthful hope and idealism, there did come a time in my life when I felt discouraged, demoralised and cynical. My work felt meaningless and I even considered giving up medical practice. I had lost my way. One day I shared my malaise with an understanding friend who responded by reading me the following Zen story. I thought about its sharp wisdom for a long time – and carried on.

> There was a certain army doctor whose job it was to accompany soldiers to battle and tend to their wounds on the battlefield. But it seemed like every time he patched someone up, the soldier would just go right back into battle and end up being wounded again, or killed. After this had happened over and over again, the doctor finally broke down.
>
> 'If it is their fate to die, why should I try to save them? And if my medicine means anything, then why do they go back to war to get killed?'
>
> Not understanding what significance there was in being an army doctor, he felt extremely confused and could not carry on with his work. So he went up into the mountains in search of a Master. After studying with a Zen Master for some time, he finally understood his problem and de-scended back down the mountain to continue his practice.
>
> Thereafter, whenever he was troubled with doubts, he simply said, 'Because I am a doctor.' (Chung 1994, p.42–43)

While travelling through life, I have been privileged to meet many remarkable people: Egyptian adepts, Tibetan lamas, shamans in Peru, Buddhist monks in Thailand, an avatar in Germany, gurus in India, teachers in America, philosophers and contemplative nuns in England. I have learnt something from all of them of a conscious stillness behind the world of appearances. The teaching of advaita, meaning 'not two', points beyond the divisions of the restless, separate ego, to the unchanging reality of a supreme consciousness that universally lights us all. To realise that the consciousness of our deepest being is not different from that, is said to be the aim and end of spiritual endeavour. Some have simply called it 'waking up' to who we really are.

And on those difficult days, which we all have when facing people seeking help, when I sometimes think it would be much easier not to have to listen to the message in the pain, but instead prescribe a drug to 'take it away', I continue to learn that in accepting and working positively with 'what is', both 'good' and 'bad', lies our gradual enlightenment: the greatest of all healing virtues. Because in the end, shining in wholeness, behind the distortions of disease, and woven through the laws of necessity and fate – as the substance holding everything together – love turns out to be who we really are. And everyone knows it because who, in the end, is not passionate about the truth of love?

References

Chung, T.C. (1994) *Zen Speaks – Shouts of Nothingness.* London: Aquarian. Translateb by Brian Bruya.

Dixon, D., Sweeney, K. and Pereira Gray, D. (1999) 'The physician healer: Ancient magic and modern science?' *British Journal of General Practice 49*, 441, 309–312.

Dubos, R.J. (1999) *So Human an Animal: How we are shaped by surroundings and events.* New York: Harper.

Guardian, The (2003) 'The Great Drugs Lottery.' 9 December, p.14.

Haehl, R. (2001) *Samuel Hahnemann. His Life and Work.* Vol. 1. New Delhi: B. Jain Publishers.

Hahnemann, S. (1982) *Organon of Medicine.* 5th & 6th edition. New Dehli: B. Jain Publishers. Translated by R.E. Dudgeon.

Illich, I. (1974) *Limits to Medicine. Medical Nemesis: The Exploration of Health.* London: Marion Boyars.

Jung, C.G. (1969) 'The Archetype of the Collective Unconscious.' In *Collected Works of C.G. Jung, Vol. 9, Part I.* Princeton: Princeton University Press. Translated by R.F.C. Hull.

Jung, C.G. (1982) 'Late Thoughts.' In *Memories, Dreams and Reflections.* Edited by Aniela Jaffe. Glasgow: Williams Collins Sons Ltd.

Kent, J.T. (1979) *Kent's Lectures on Homeopathic Philosophy.* London: Thorsens Ltd.

Launer, J. (2003) 'Narrative-based medicine: A passing fad or a giant leap for general practice?' *British Journal of General Practice, 53,* 487, 91–92.

Lazarou, J.L., Pomeranz, B.H. and Corey, M.P.N. 'Incidence of adverse drug reactions in hospitalized patients; A meta-analysis of prospective studies.' *Journal of the American Medical Association, 279,* 1200–5.

Linde, K., Clausius, N., Ramirez, G., Melchart, D., Eitel, F., Hedges, L.V. and Jonas, W.B. (1997) 'Are the clinical effects of homoeopathy placebo effects? A meta-analysis of placebo-controlled trials.' *The Lancet, 350,* 834–843.

Lockie, A. (1989) *The Family Guide to Homeopathy. The Safe Form of Medicine for the Future.* London: Hamish Hamilton Ltd.

Luthe, W. and Schultz, J. (1969) *Vol. 1, Autogenic Methods. Vol. 2, Medical Applications. Vol. 3, Applications in Psychotherapy, Vol. 4, Research and Theory. Vol. 5, Dynamics of Autogenic Neutralisation. Vol. 6, Treatment with Autogenic Neutralisation.* New York: Grune & Stratton Inc.

Maride, Y., Haramburu, F., Requejo, A.A., Begaud, B. (1997) 'Under-reporting of adverse drug reactions in general practice.' *British Journal of Clinical Pharmacology, 43,* 177–181.

Mihajlov, M. (1976) 'Mystical Experience of the Labour Camps.' In *Kontinent 2: The Alternative Voice of Russia and Eastern Europe.* Edited by Alexander Solzhenitysn. London: Coronet Books and Andre Deutsch.

Paterson, C., and Britten, N. (1999) 'Doctors can't help much: The search for an alternative.' *British Journal of General Practice 49,* 445, 626–629.

Pirmohamed, M., James, S., Meakin, S., Green, C., Scott, A., Walley, T., *et al.* (2004) 'Adverse drug reactions as a cause of admission to hospital: Prospective analysis of 18, 820 patients.' *British Medical Journal, 329,* 15–19.

Reilly, D., Taylor, M. and Beattie, N. (1994) 'Is evidence for homeopathy reproducible?' *The Lancet, 344*, 1601–1606.

Schmidt, J.M. (1996) 'Anthropology and medicine.' *British Homeopathic Journal 82*, 288–296.

Sharma, P.V. (1999) *Sushruta Samhita*. Vol. 1. India: Chaukhambha Visvabharti.

Smith, K.R. (1976) *The Gurdjieff Work*. London: Turnstone Books.

Swayne, J. (2000) *International Directory of Homeopathy*. London: Churchill Livingstone.

Viksveen, P. (2003) 'Antibiotics and the development of resistant microorganisms. Can homeopathy be an alternative?' *Homeopathy, 92*, 99–107.

World Health Organisation (1998) *The Global Burden of Disease and Injury*. Geneva: World Health Organisation.

Further reading

Bennet, J.G. (1973) *Gurdjieff: Making a New World*. London: Turnstone Books.

Coulter, H.L. (1973) *Divided Legacy – The Conflict Between Homeopathy and the American Medical Association*. California: North Atlantic Books.

IMT Nuremberg (1947–49) *Trials of the Major War Criminals before the International Military Tribunal* (42 vols.). Nuremberg: IMT.

Jung, C.G. (1984) 'Paracelsus the Physician.' In *The Spirit in Man, Art and Literature*. Ark Paperbacks. Translated by R.E.C. Hull.

Richardson-Boedler, C. (1999) 'The Doctrine of Signatures: A historical, philosophical and scientific view.' *British Homeopathic Journal, 88*, 172–177.

Introduction to Chapter 3

David Owen, perhaps more than any other writer in this book, wants to understand the psychology of the medical profession, its power structures and emotional repression which he sees as potentially, and sometimes actually, harmful. His story challenges us to examine some of our core beliefs about such issues as the emotional support of doctors, and how emotional repression is built into the profession. His wish is to bring the heart back into medicine.

David writes, 'Healing the wounds of the profession is something about which I am passionate,' and he is honest enough to know that that includes his own wounds. I asked him what was the most important message he would like the reader to take away from his writing and he replied:

> The most important thing a reader will get from this chapter is insight into how, for one doctor, their view of themselves and their profession changed by reflection about themselves and looking inside.

Chapter 3

Medicine – A Suitable Case for Treatment?
David Owen

My father was a medical doctor. He worked long hours as a general practitioner, as did my mother in bringing up four young children. Despite their busyness there was a lot of love in the family but in common with most families a lot of different needs. Looking back, from an early age, like many second born children, I was attracted to the role of referee in our house. In my wish to keep the peace and by trying to prevent normal family conflicts I was giving myself power in the family.

For several years, we lived above the surgery where medicine and family life intermingled. My father worked from his heart giving his all to patients. He often talked about patients and work. It gave him a great deal, but I am not sure he felt adequately acknowledged for all his efforts. The health care system seemed to keep asking for more and more and was never satisfied. Although we were relatively well off, it never felt to me that his caring was, financially, fairly rewarded. Even so, the grateful patient, occasional thank you or small present meant more than any payment. I enjoyed going with him now and again to visit patients and became aware of the privilege it was to belong to the medical profession, something I still feel. But I started to ask the question then, and have continued to do so, about how emotionally supported doctors are by our profession and how clear our contract is with our patients.

It was in these early stages of my life that the personality traits I now recognise in myself started to develop. I would like to share something about these traits and how they were formed with you, in the wish that the universal aspects as well as the personal ones might help you to reflect on your own.

The first of these traits that I noticed was the one that began 'watching'; observing not just what happened physically but most importantly the emotions to which I was sensitive, in order to detect and anticipate changes in the emotional atmosphere around me. I did this partly to be on guard, and partly from a sense of responsibility. I found myself looking out wherever possible to manage my own and others' conflict. My parents had moved away from their friends and family and as a consequence of this, there were not many others who could look out for them and like other children I watched out for them.

Although my childhood was emotionally charged, it was as part of a supportive but challenging family and certainly far from those traumatic experiences of childhood that I later witnessed in many of my patients. I have often wondered just how they cope. For myself growing up, because of my extreme sensitivity and sense of responsibility, I would try to make family life and relationships, especially difficult situations, into a game. This is where my psychological quality as a 'game player' developed, in order to protect myself. I realised while playing certain games in competition with my brothers and sister that the price of being the winner meant that there had to be a loser, and that this upset at losing could sometimes be even greater than the satisfaction of winning. Soon afterwards I realised that, whenever I lost at anything, I could minimise the pain and hurt by telling myself it was 'only a game'. This simple technique of reducing and avoiding pain by diminishing its significance has allowed me to empathise with others' pain without taking it too personally. I see many patients doing this too, by saying 'It's only a cold', or 'A funny/strange thing happened to me'. The opposite is also true: that in some situations patients will magnify the pain with the opposite story – it has to be serious, e.g. 'It's arthritis', 'It's cancer', 'It's killing me'.

At about age seven I remember feeling that one or two teachers took a deeper, more personal interest in me and supported and encouraged me, which played a large part in my awakening. I started learning about the wider world and began to realise what a wonderful place it was. These qualities of support and encouragement I try to emulate in my own work, especially in teaching others. I loved to listen to people telling me stories about the world. If ever I heard a sense of wonder in the storyteller's voice, usually based on their personal experience, my attention was immediately engaged. One side of me was particularly fascinated by being the focus of attention, whether being asked a question or taking part in the school plays. At the same time, another side of me was acutely anxious, and very sensitive to being seen. Looking back, I now know that whenever I was being closely observed in anything like a critical light, it closed me down and created a huge amount of tension, which sat with me and led to anxiety. It has only been gaining insight into my own anxiety that has allowed me to help others with theirs.

At the age of eight or nine, along with many other children, I started to create a fantasy world around me. I could escape into this alternative world whenever I was feeling unhappy or sad – or indeed, use it when I wanted to impress others, since I soon realised the magical power of weaving stories. And so the 'storyteller' developed in me. Through this part of me, I learnt to know the difference between when people were showing me who they really were at the deepest level, and when they were telling stories to protect themselves. I have found that people will often hide behind their stories, but there are always links to their reality and, with permission, sensitivity and a sense of exploration, the deepest aspects of people's lives are invariably waiting to surface.

By the time I was 11, I was clearly having some struggle with language skills, and around this time, was diagnosed as having dyslexia. I remember telling myself that this was only someone else's diagnosis, but deep down I felt a sense of failure. This led to two things: first, a determination to succeed in my own way and second, permission to work in other ways. It raised my emotional sensitivity to a higher degree. I was rapidly developing what has later come to be called emotional intelligence.

When I was 13, I went away to a boarding school two or three hours' drive from my home. I was bullied in the first term, seriously enough to know what it felt like to be a victim. And although I started to explore my own sense of failure and rejection that might have attracted this bullying, it still took a great deal from friends, some teachers and myself to rekindle the feeling of self-worth that had been undermined by this process.

Attending an all-boys school has obviously had a huge effect on my emotional development and, like many adolescents, much of the expression of my emotions in puberty was through the world of fantasy. Many of these factors led to a split within me: for example, into the polarities between home and school, failure and success, happiness and sadness, confidence and lack of confidence. Fortunately, I soon found that I was able to relate to a wide variety of people, and could befriend both the most successful in the peer group and the underdog.

I started to trust the teachers, who in turn trusted me to achieve in their subjects. For example, the chemistry teacher, who did a lot to build my confidence, particularly inspired me. Trust was important to me then, and still is, especially because the different models of the world that I was being taught in the sciences kept being eroded. I remember being told that atoms were 'it', then electrons were 'it', then quarks were 'it'; each of these was sold as a 'final' truth, only to find later that they were inaccurate. I can't believe that the benefits of teaching such simplistic models outweigh the distrust generated in the students both about their subject and their teacher. Perhaps this is why I am a passionate teacher of how I see it, but the downside may be that I don't know when to stop. It was at this point that I became aware of the split between the scientist and the artist within me. I pursued the sciences, but with a strong emotional and artistic presence. It was becoming clear to me that by exploring this paradox – of the two different worlds portrayed by science and art – I would also be exploring something of my own inner state.

In an attempt to address the questions that the tension between science and art raised, I felt drawn to studying medicine. I thought it would bring together the science of how things work and the art of relating to people. The artist in me felt born to this as a vocation, but I was aware that the scientist was perhaps educated into it.

So, after the exams and a year growing up, it was off to London to medical school. That first year was quite an experience. The approach to the training of medical students where I studied seemed both to focus on making students feel 'special' (possibly because of the high acaedemic entry requirements) and to overwhelm us with factual information and memory tasks. This led me, and I suspect many others, to feel that whatever we did we could not completely belong in the world outside of medicine. However, despite arriving full of positive intentions, I resisted immersing myself completely within the medical school environment, perhaps because of the lack of reflective or critical thinking taking place there.

The 'person' I saw most of was the cadaver that we were dissecting. In the first term we dissected out the legs and arms, in the second, the thorax and abdomen, and by the third term, the head. Our cadaver was ritually – sorry – surgically, pulled apart by eight of us. Is it any wonder that doctors are susceptible to problems with values? Fundamentally, I experienced it as an abusive process but then perhaps, in a way, all education and socialisation is. Here were some of the most intelligent minds in the country learning the name for every muscle, nerve, vein and artery in the body. I was initially surprised, then disappointed, at not being encouraged to think for myself, but instead having to focus on learning facts. The education wasn't so much about acquiring knowledge (although that was the overt agenda) but was, on reflection, an initiation into the 'medical club'.

The benefits of strong bonds between fellow members were obvious even at medical school. What was strange to me was the lack of a culture of questioning and challenging by students and juniors in the profession, possibly, I now realise, due to the career progression by patronage. This has, I believe, led to the values and objectives of the medical profession (some of which I explore later) remaining unchallenged and I suspect mainly unconscious. I wonder if this plays a part in society's questioning of its relationship with the medical profession, including the movement to alternatives, and why there is less trust and the wish for external checks, including questioning the basis of self-regulation.

In many ways I felt I had failed to sit comfortably in either the medical club or the outside world and the struggle to reconcile these left me in a lonely place. As a result of this, part of me still remains passionate about helping students feel a sense of belonging while they are training. When a health professional has experienced this in their training, I believe they are more likely to know what is required to hold and support patients while they are being treated. Creating organisational structures that can foster the individual, whether he or she is giving or receiving the training or treatment, is a challenge for all of us involved in health care.

Medical education has moved on thanks to many sensitive and caring individuals contributing to it, but at the time examining values was not part of our curriculum and many of our feelings about training and practice were never explored. My experience is that feelings we repress such as frustration, anxiety and uncertainty surface later as symptoms. I wonder how much the stress that doctors find themselves under is a result of having to repress so much of themselves in their training and work. Certainly, by looking at these things I have found my satisfaction with work has improved greatly. Without this insight I believe it is easy to set up an abusive process where a more powerful organisation can take advantage of less powerful individuals.

Those abuses within the medical system, so often reported in the media of late, can perhaps be understood in one way as symptoms of the sickness within the profession, and not necessarily aberrant acts. Most doctors reading about one or other medical colleague being investigated will probably if they are honest, think, 'There, but for the grace of God, go I.'

For the medical profession to address these issues meaningfully we need to see this behaviour as an expression of our collective behaviour, even if it is only being acted out by a few individuals. I believe we need to understand the psychological reasons for it, and consciously to begin to work through the issues. I think this is the real and pressing development issue facing the medical profession, not just keeping up to date with the latest technological advances. For example, the fear of consultants and of passing exams felt by students seems to model a way of working that resonates to the fear of failure or litigation that permeates much of the medical profession.

During the summer holidays, at the end of my first year at medical school, I joined a tight-knit meditation group. I knew, without a doubt, that I needed to do some work on finding out more about myself and what was real in the world. I also received huge insights from this journey. The requirements of the group gave me a strong sense of belonging, not dissimilar to my experiences in boarding school. It provided a 'safe place' from the outer and medical worlds, a place where I could explore the inner work that I needed to do in order to reconcile myself with the world that I was facing. You can imagine the split in me between these two worlds and therefore the challenge to my keeping this contemplative life and medical school together. Being so engrossed in the pathology of the world while trying to practise sensitively fascinated me.

It felt like a huge privilege to me when I was introduced to my first patients as a medical student. The contract is different from any other relationship you, or they, are likely to have. Our patients showed us everything of themselves. It was a place where they no longer had to hide, and there was time to hear their life's story: a privilege. For me, the dreams and fantasies I had of how the world might be for other people were shattered as I heard frequent and recurrent stories of suffering and pain.

The stark reality of the suffering most people experience could be responded to in two different ways: either to shut down, or to seek a meaning for it, something I did by retreating within myself. Some medical students survive by shutting down. A few 'go in search of meaning', whether through a reflective process or specialisation in a microcosm of their world. All find their way of adjusting to sitting with patients' distress. How well we come to terms with the distress we see is, I think, crucial to how well doctors survive in this system. Some detach from the reality of the distress, becoming voyeurs of others life experiences; some take it out on 'juniors' or at home; others begin to resent their patients or minimise their suffering.

The more I explored the meaning of illness, the more I found patients would tell me their whole story. It was and is surprising how ready people are to reveal themselves. It also surprised me how therapeutic patients found this, and how grateful they were. I wanted to understand what made people tick, where they were going, and how their illnesses were related to what was happening in their lives. This sometimes brought me into conflict with my teachers.

It was hearing these patients' stories that was my initiation into doctoring. Not just by looking down the microscope at a body specimen or attending post-mortems, or putting my hands inside people's anaesthetised bodies during operations. Not surprisingly, my relationship with the world shifted, and shifted to such a degree that it does not strike me as strange now that some of the greatest social revolutionaries have been and are doctors. Nor does it strike me as strange that doctors can commit acts of both tremendous cruelty as well as tremendous compassion.

It seems strange to relate to patients in so many challenging ways without explicit support or occasionally reflecting on the issues and feelings raised. For example, I wonder if it is possible to be able to conduct regular vaginal or penile examinations without raising questions about the nature of sexual relationships. Nor does it seem possible to see a fungating breast mass, cr to carry out a surgical mastectomy, without questioning the fundamental nurturing role of the breast. I could never sit with someone in great pain, nor watch someone die without reflecting on the purpose of life. The body and its parts can have their shadow side revealed in stark ways, and if carers do not have a forum for expressing and working through the feelings generated by working with them, there is a likelihood of increasing levels of emotional reperession which can later surface as burn-out symptoms.

I could not see people die in all those different ways without needing to ask what life and death was all about. And because what was happening during my training and early experience as a doctor was not made conscious, I internalised my feelings including the pain – and sometimes even felt in some way guilty and responsible for what was happening to patients. Is it any wonder we have so many doctors who are 'wounded healers'? I certainly was one of those who felt driven to help others. But behind the white coat, the stethoscope or the medical credentials this wound is, I believe, at the centre of what drives the medical profession. It is no wonder that until the 'drivers' are made conscious, the medical system will struggle for clarity about its direction.

It was with great relief that I discovered what is now called complementary medicine. At that time in the UK it was considered to be just many unrelated alternatives to orthodox medical practice. I chose to study both acupuncture and homeopathy (although they were not widely known or accepted at that time) as a medical student because they offered different models of care and had an interesting philosophical basis. During my fifth medical year I visited India and Sri

Lanka to study these and also regularly attended outpatient clinics at the Homeopathic Hospital in London. It surprised and intrigued me to find this was, and still is, an NHS hospital, and a place where I realised others who questioned some of the dominant orthodox thinking could find a place to work. As a medical student I did a lot of 'sitting-in' at various orthodox outpatient departments to see how diseases were managed. Not a lot was mentioned, or taught, about how people could heal themselves. During my time there I would feel people's pulses (in a new way, according to the Chinese system of medicine I was learning), and try to classify which homeopathic groups they belonged to (in homeopathy we classify patients with chronic disease into miasmatic groups). I became even more intrigued about patients' stories of what had happened to them both before and after they became ill. I realised that people's illnesses were very much a part of their story and that their illness, even if unpleasant, often had meaning to them. Even though most just wanted to be rid of their symptoms (and the medical system tried hard to do this in some way), I began to realise that many people needed their illnesses and had something to learn from them before they could start to recover fully.

As I gradually became more interested in the different therapies, I would needle various different acupuncture points on my own body to see what effect it had on me. I would also take homeopathic remedies in potency to see if I could detect which part of my body they were affecting, and how. By the end of my time at medical school I was ambivalent about qualifying because I was unsure about what would come next. I might have been trained but I was emotionally not ready to work with patients. I was aware of what I did not want to do and was fortunate to be able to re-examine fundamentally how it is possible to work with patients by training in homeopathy.

There followed a year's 'apprenticeship' as a junior hospital doctor doing medicine and surgery. When I was looking after a patient, I wanted to be able to really get to know them as an individual, and concentrate on their particular pattern of illness. The time available and organisation often prevented this. This first year is for most doctors a transforming time and for some a brutal time. I learnt about responsibility, a strange hierarchy from patients to colleagues and 'the profession' and above all, to my patron and boss. I learnt about where patients go when they are ill and the personal and institutional fear of death that pervades medicine. I became interested in the power of teams, and how institutions working under great pressure are set up and maintained. I realised that, while it was important to think of the big picture and address questions like who should get what care when, it was impossible to meet everyone's needs. There would never be a time when the last patient was cured.

I left knowing that to work with patients as I wanted to it would be in a health care system that would look very different from the hospital one. I realised that, while many carers blame the system for limiting the type and amount of care they can give, from another perspective, if you really want to give that sort of holistic care, you can create a system to deliver it. This has been my challenge and is, I believe, the challenge of the medical profession generally.

Part of what inhibited me (and still inhibits the profession) was a fear of failure or of making a mistake. Once, after a particularly long day, during a time when I was working every third night and weekend, in addition to my normal daytime job, I was awoken yet again in the very early hours by the shrill sound of my pager going off. When I answered the call, I was asked to return (for the fourth time that night) to the ward. Instead of getting up there and then, due to exhaustion, I fell back to sleep. When I was paged again half an hour later, the patient's condition had deteriorated significantly, and I arrived too late to make a difference. I immediately felt a sense of failure and lack of worth. I felt alone with this and while I know now that most 'apprentices' feel something like this at some time, I didn't know it then. I can see now that this is a big factor in why many doctors feel that they can never do enough to help, and then project their resentment onto patients. The failure of the profession to help me work through or support me with this feeling is, I believe, at the heart of the low morale within the medical profession. It explains why many doctors feel they are being taken advantage of, and also why they can be manipulated.

The other way some doctors cope with such failure is by making it something of a credential: the worst thing that happened that you got away with. It leaves you with a fear of being found out. No wonder the profession closes ranks and becomes secretive. The credential ties you into the system, through shame and guilt. While this dynamic remains unconscious, the pattern can only repeat itself. The abused become the abusers. It was through reflection and meditation that I began to develop insight into what was happening to me.

I started to understand it was not only the doctors who set the values and culture of their profession, but also the patients. In many situations patients expect and encourage doctors to behave in certain ways. I believe patients and doctors must each accept some responsibility for how the other behaves. You don't have an expert unless people give up their own expertise.

By the time I had completed a year in hospitals, I realised that the contract I wished to have with patients was to help them get themselves better, not to 'do something' to them. I knew that I wanted to become a homeopathic physician because it allowed me to work in this way. I also welcomed the chance to meet and study with other doctors similarly questioning their way forward. For me, becoming a homeopathic doctor allowed me to bring together the different qualities and sides of my personality. It was the first time I felt 'at home' professionally.

Homeopathy is uniquely placed between the medical and the psychodynamic models of health, and can provide a truly holistic view of individuals, their illnesses and their treatment. It enables me to work with people who are suffering while focusing on the questions I know are important for the patient and myself to answer: not just what is wrong but why a patient might need a particular illness and what must happen so that they no longer need it. The ability homeopathy has to allow this way of looking at illness – as an opportunity to grow – has always remained important to me, and is why I am committed to its practice and teaching.

It was an interesting experience to put a brass plate up in a room and start a practice from scratch. In the first week I had two patients. As you can imagine, those early patients got a lot of attention from me, perhaps even too much, but it was a fantastic way to learn. I immersed myself in homeopathy. My practice built steadily and, for a while, my homeopathic approach was just grafted onto my basic medical training. Over time I started to develop my own approach to working holistically as I realised there were limitations to the homeopathic approach. I explored other complementary therapies because, through them, I found other parts of the jigsaw puzzle I needed in order to work holistically. I learnt about hypnotherapy, nutritional medicine, allergy and environmental medicine, and osteopathic manipulation.

I envisioned establishing a holistic general practice using complementary treatment for all comers, but realised that, at that time, not everyone might be ready for a holistic approach.

For some patients it was exactly what they wanted, but for many others, 'seeing the doctor' was still about handing over responsibility. They were not yet willing or able to take responsibility for their own health.

In those early days of practice, I realised there were many limitations in the historic texts of homeopathy and so, looking at what was useful and what was not, I started to re-write them in my own mind. While acknowledging the many excellent contributions made to the subject by different homeopaths over the years, nevertheless, I found myself resisting the tendency to make 'gurus' of the various teachers. I would frequently reflect on inconsistencies or limits to my knowledge and often found synchronicity would deliver a training course, a patient or a book that offered insights into the difficulties. Not uncommonly, I realised it was often the way that I was looking at the problem, or what I was unrealistically expecting of myself, that was causing the problem.

Professionally, this was an exciting but lonely time in my life. Luckily, my relationship with my wife, Sue, bloomed at this time and nourished me. It was this sense of professional isolation that led me to attend training events and meetings with other complementary therapists. I became involved in the work of the Faculty of Homeopathy, a professional body for homeopathic health professionals recognised around the world. After some years, I was elected President and enjoyed the chance to explore organisationally how to address representing, supporting and facilitating the development of individuals in a profession. I had the chance to recognise the very real difficulties of 'doing it differently'. I could revisit the indulgent ideals of the naïve apprentice and see that to do it differently requires a willingness to change, a great deal of time to reflect on the issues and the clear realisation that a profession is just the sum of its individual members.

It soon became apparent to me that many therapists I knew, including practitioners in complementary and alternative medicine, tried to 'hunt the right remedy' in their clinical cases. When this did not work they would berate themselves for failing, just as I had done. So it was a wonderful revelation for me to find a like-minded colleague in Dr Lee Holland, a consultant psychiatrist who had also retrained and was practising as a homeopathic physician. Together we discussed our difficult cases, realising that it was precisely our difficult cases that could teach us so much more than our successful ones. This led me to adopt several models of how homeopathy could be applied in different situations, but always based on the principle of finding 'the centre of the case', which relates to the reason why a patient needs a particular set of symptoms at that particular time.

While I was exploring the best way to find the centre of disturbance, I noticed that I was becoming less 'present' as a listener in some difficult consultations. I might withdraw when things got tough, or become overly intellectual. I recognised this as a pattern I used when emotions started to surface. A breakthrough for me was when I started to trust what I myself was feeling when sitting opposite patients, and gradually I learnt how to make use of what I felt. It almost invariably had some relevance to the case and enabled me to empathise more closely with my patients. My whole scientific and medical training had discouraged me from engaging emotionally. It was only as I began to use my emotional intelligence consciously that it became possible to really start working with my patients' deeper levels of need and hurt.

It was this feeling that there was a better way of working that led me to join a small group of colleagues to talk about running a homeopathic teaching course. Initially, our vision was to teach postgraduate homeopathy, to teach what we were learning. However, it was clear that to do this, the students would have to be well grounded in homeopathic principles and philosophy, and also be open to a reflective style of learning. This involves a training style that recognises that real learning happens not just by the acquisition of facts but also by entering into a process of growth. In order to do this we started a course in homeopathic education, run by ourselves as the Homeo-pathic Physicians Teaching Group (HPTG). The guiding principle, placed right at the centre of the course, was the importance of self-discovery in any learning process. For this to take place, participants needed to be able to trust their teachers and feel supported in confronting their own lack of knowledge. It has been truly amazing to see the changes health professionals have made to themselves and their approach to treatment. One doctor commented, 'I've started to enjoy seeing patients again', another that 'The course has changed my life.' The message from participants is invariably that it's fun, challenging, stimulating and very worthwhile. The friendship with teachers and students on the course has been the biggest positive experience of my career and the most important things I have learnt from the HPTG is that training requires support, education and development and that the outcome is trans-formational for both participants and teachers.

Healing the wounds of the profession is something about which I am passionate. For me, this is not a matter of learning something new, but more about re-connecting with who we are. I feel these same lessons and opportunities can be made available through a structure of reflection and supervision for all health carers. This is, I believe, necessary not only to allow patients to be seen as whole people, but also for the sake of the doctors' own well being. It is only when this shift in attitude has grown and developed, mirrored by changes to our professional organisations, that doctors will, I believe, really be able to feel they are supported by and belong to these organisations, to come in from their professional isolation and be fully part of a team.

I truly believe that doctors coming together and working co-operatively and openly can, in time, change the whole way medicine is practised. I cannot see any new discovery or external fix ever working in this transformative way. There is an opportunity for all of us to challenge the old orthodox ways of thinking, and to start discovering some of these inner truths about ourselves. As a way of clarifying and bringing the values and insights of my personal life into focus, supervision and being a part of a support team of teachers and students in HPTG has been invaluable. My great interest now in taking part in supervision groups for homeopaths and other health carers is due to my belief that this is where our personal development can be supported, our clinical practice improved, and where the health profession of the future will emerge. The personal, clinical and organisational are not seperate, but in fact, complement one another.

Introducing reflective practice and supervision into the centre of our professional work is my passion, and I believe that by doing this there are ample opportunities here to balance and influence the way medicine is practised. Of course, this opportunity to change is resisted by many, and it may be that the profession has to move still further away from a person-centred approach before doctors and patients really start to seek out opportunities to change. To a seasoned homeopath, these are all just symptoms of the deeper underlying disturbance, waiting to be recognised and healed. Perhaps now is the time to 'find the centre of the case'?

Introduction to Chapter 4

In this piece, Peter Gregory, a veterinary surgeon, describes his love of nature and through this introduces us to the plant and mineral connections to homeopathic remedies. His wish to understand the healing power of homeopathy has led him to quantum physics for an explanation. His observations about the connections between owner and animal add an extra dimension to the question of the origins and cures of illness.

When I asked Peter what was the most important message he would like the reader to take away from his writing, he replied:

> I would like them to realise how homeopathy challenges our perceptions, and how its study can lead us to a deeper understanding of how our universe operates.

Chapter 4

Seeking the True Nature
Peter Gregory

I was born and raised in Sheffield, in what is now South Yorkshire. The prosperity of Sheffield was built around the manufacture of cutlery and of steel. The heart of the heavy industry was the valley of the River Don, which rises in the hills of the Peak District, runs through the centre of the city, and then heads eastwards through Rotherham and Doncaster towards the sea, and even in my childhood enormous quantities of steel were produced there. It was in Sheffield that Ibbotson made his chance discovery of stainless steel, when he noticed that a discarded piece of metal on a pile of refuse had not corroded in the same way as the rest. My grandfather was chief metallurgist at the Parkgate Iron and Steel Company and later at Edgar Allen's, both major producers in their time, particularly of special steels. Sheffield still produces large tonnages of these, despite the decline in the industry as a whole. In between these times my grandfather lectured in metallurgy at Sheffield University and worldwide. With such a powerful family influence it is not surprising that as a child I developed an interest in rocks and minerals and indeed, for a long time, I intended to become a geologist.

Despite its industry, Sheffield is an extremely pleasant city. The steep valleys which in the 18th century provided the water power for the cutlery industry were abandoned as steam power came into vogue and the industry moved down to the lower reaches of the Don. These valleys now provide pleasant wooded walks past disused mill ponds, from the open moors of the Peak District right down to within a mile of the city centre so that wherever one may be in the city, it is always possible to see some greenery.

Shortly after the Second World War, during which so much of the centre of the city was devastated in the blitz, the city limits were extended to cater for new housing development. The border between Yorkshire and Derbyshire, which before that had represented the boundary between the ancient kingdoms of Mercia and Northumbria, was moved westwards by a few miles to encompass not only the two small Derbyshire villages of Dore and Totley, but a considerable area of open moorland as well. The latter was continuous with that mass of wilderness which now bears the name 'The Dark Peak', and it was around this time that the Peak District itself was recognised as an entity and declared as the nation's first National Park.

When I was six months old, my family – father, mother, an older brother and myself – moved from our terraced house near the centre of the city to a new semi-detached in a cul-de-sac in Dore. Despite the new housing (which by modern standards was a very modest development indeed), Dore still retained its village atmosphere, and one of the joys of being brought up there was its rural setting.

My mother loved nature and from her I learned to appreciate the wild flowers that grew in abundance in the meadows around the village and in the woods and moors which were so easily accessible from our home. When I was old enough to do so, I spent many hours and days exploring the countryside in the company of my dog. Ah yes, the dogs! We always had a dog. The first was Kim, a Scottie cross, the result of a mismating of my grandmother's Scottie bitch with an unknown Rotherham vagrant. I remember his tricky nature and his abhorrence of bathing, which he expressed violently one day after rolling in something horrible on a walk. My mother's battle with him left her in need of stitches in a hand wound. In his old age he developed cancer and was put to sleep by the local vet. We were then without a dog for a little while, until grandfather's doctor's Cocker Spaniel bitch had puppies and on one of our regular trips to my grandfather's bungalow in Rotherham, we were presented with a small golden bundle of fur. Rather predictably, we immediately named him 'Rusty'.

Rusty soon became my dog, rather than the family's pet. I was ten, and perhaps just old enough to take some responsibility for him. True, my mother fed him, but I walked him. Rusty and I knew every bit of the local woods and moors. He slept on my bed and rarely left my side. We did everything right for him and he returned our care with absolute loyalty. In fact, he was sometimes a bit too loyal. Occasionally he would get on my parents' bed and guard items of clothing. Any approach was greeted with snarls and growls and I have no doubt he would have followed up with serious violence if pushed. In a vain attempt to gain the upper hand, my mother once took to him with my father's fishing rod; the resultant damage, along with the obvious futility of the exercise, ensured that it was not repeated. Rusty's piece de resistance was performed one evening when he would not allow the baby-sitter up the stairs to check on my brother and me. The message 'You shall not pass' was apparently very clearly expressed.

By this time my interest in geology had developed, and I took every opportunity to learn about the rocks, minerals and fossils I encountered on trips into the Peak District. This might be on family outings in the car, on picnics or on walks. The lead-mining industry of the White Peak (the limestone area in the heart of Derbyshire) had been largely defunct since well before the war, but the spoil heaps from the hundreds of small mines and shafts that pepper the area provided rich pickings for one such as me. To this day I have specimens of many of the minerals of the area: Fluor spar, Barytes and Galena, for instance, found with a minimum of fossicking on such tips. My other passion was football: playing the game myself, and watching and supporting Sheffield Wednesday, in those days one of the leading clubs in the country.

When he was three years old, Rusty caught distemper. Our vet visited regularly and treated him with all the newest antibiotics and all the supportive therapy available. Despite this, over a period of weeks he deteriorated and was put to sleep. I was completely devastated. My closest friend had left me and I can still touch the pain I felt at the time. At least it was permissible for a young boy to show his grief at the loss of his dog. Many years later, on losing another, older, canine friend, it was more difficult, though I am pleased that our society is at last beginning to recognise the reality and the enormity of the grief which losing an animal companion brings.

It was during one of the vet's visits to Rusty that I suddenly decided, at the age of 13, that I wanted to be a vet. I would like to say that this decision stemmed from a conscious desire to relieve the suffering of such poor beasts as Rusty, but I don't remember it being that way. The idea seemed to pop into my head and just felt right. However, I have no doubt that my experience with Rusty's illness was what initiated the idea. Indeed I have met many people who have decided to enter one of the healing professions as the result of suffering such a painful experience, and I wonder how common the phenomenon is.

By this time I had left the village school and was attending grammar school. I found science a little difficult and yet languages seemed to require none of the mental toil which it took to get my head round Newton's Laws or the periodic table. There would be times later on in my academic career when I seriously questioned my decision to become a vet and wondered why I had not instead become a language teacher, but more of that later. Despite these difficulties, I duly achieved the necessary A levels and, at the ridiculously young age of 17, moved on to Bristol University, leaving behind Jasper, the rather dippy Cocker Spaniel who had replaced Rusty.

Veterinary education in the late 1960s and early 1970s was uninspiring to say the least. Formal lectures were interspersed with practical sessions that were intended to provide some interest, but the atmosphere was decidedly stuffy and fear certainly pervaded my studies. This all made the experience of learning tedious. As vets we had more formal lecture time than any other faculty, and while many students threw themselves into the freedom and richness of university life, the vets lived in another world of long hours spent studying, trying desperately to assimilate the mass of information with which we were daily presented. In addition to this, examinations came fast and furious, and my overriding memory was of returning to university at the start of a new term in the knowledge that I was not going to get home again until I had sat exams.

The summer term meant degree exams: failure meant expulsion, or if you were lucky, resits which would dominate and ruin the summer vacation. It is only recently that I have managed to let go of the feeling of fear and indignation that the smell of newly mown grass used to trigger, and I still occasionally dream that I have to take finals again, with no warning and no chance to prepare adequately. I developed a huge feeling of indignation that others could so affect my life. As anyone who has endured the stress and repressed anger of a veterinary education will affirm, there is a point, or several points in the five years, where one reassesses the decision, and considers an alternative career. I always had immense admiration for those few who actually had the courage to step off the treadmill and develop different skills. It was far easier to take the course of least resistance and soldier on – and of course it would be worth it in the end, wouldn't it? (Two years after graduation, being roused from sleep at 3am to deliver a calf in a freezing barn on top of the moors, the answer was definitely 'No'.) It was at these times that the idea of learning a foreign language and teaching English overseas seemed so attractive.

In addition to the fear of failure itself there was the fear of being seen as not good enough; having to face the family, my friends and their families within the village if I dropped out. The antithesis to these feelings of inadequacy was the professional arrogance with which I was imbued. The inference at university was that by the end of the course I would know, or at least have been taught, everything there was to know about disease in animals and its treatment. With such omniscience, if as a vet I couldn't fix it then obviously no one else could. And if anyone claimed they could they were obviously lying. While other therapies were not mentioned by name, it was easy to recognise them once we were qualified; basically anyone treating animals with no formal veterinary qualification was a charlatan. This did not quite fit with the restricted Materia Medica with which we were equipped. Even in such an indoctrinated state, I was perplexed and slightly amused to find that a lecture on a viral disease such as canine distemper consisted of several paragraphs on the viral agent itself and its effects on the animal, with one or two lines devoted to the treatment. This usually consisted of antibiotics with or without corticosteroids or vitamin supplements. Occasionally fluid therapy was indicated. It was with such a narrow view of veterinary medicine that I qualified in 1972.

My first job was in Sheffield with the same 'family vets' who had ministered to Rusty and his successor. It was a mixed practice whose farming clientele were spread over an area that extended from the Yorkshire Pennines in the north to the vales of the Derbyshire Peak District in the south west. The countryside was spectacular and the work satisfying but sometimes gruelling. I suppose I caught the last few years of the 'James Herriot' lifestyle before it all but disappeared into a world of commerce and large commercial concerns. On the small animal side I began to realise how little I really knew. Aided by one of the partners, my first bitch spey was performed without fatality, despite the uncontrollable shaking of my hands; the subsequent ones required the assistance of the head 'nurse' (there were no formal qualifications in those days) who I soon found knew more about surgery than I did. Though I enjoyed surgery, there was always the fear that something would go wrong and my patient would die, and this constant fear of making a mistake and its consequences pervaded my experience of veterinary practice. And there were the night calls – calvings, colics, milk fevers and vomiting dogs. One night in four on duty, and rarely a night went by without a callout somewhere. Then back to work in the morning. One weekend on, one weekend off. For the first two years I lived in the practice house in Hillsborough, close enough to Sheffield Wednesday's football stadium to hear the roar of the crowd on match days, often as I worked in the garden, waiting for the phone to ring to call me to the next emergency. Fortunately, I was a good enough player to retain my place in Totley's village football team, despite only being available every second Saturday.

Shortly after I started work, 'Big Ears' came into my life. He was a black and white terrier cross puppy who had been abandoned at the surgery with a fractured hip. Big Ears became my constant companion. I took him to Australia when I emigrated in 1977 and I brought him back when I returned to the UK seven years later. He had an interesting life, and his veterinary history is no less colourful. In the area of North Queensland where I lived the climate was tropical and ideal for the survival of insects, snakes and arthropods such as spiders and ticks. Fleas and ticks were a continual problem to the domestic dogs, and skin allergies were one of the most frequent conditions we had to treat. Big Ears developed this problem not long after his release from three months' quarantine. Apart from weekly dips in organophosphorus insecticides to control parasites, the only treatment available was the injection of long-acting corticosteroids. As Big Ears became more resistant to the drugs, so I had to increase the dosage and each time I injected him he developed a raging thirst, extreme hunger, and the pot belly associated with the Cushingoid syndrome so well recognised as a sequel to overdosage of corticosteroids. 'There must be another way,' I thought, but I didn't know where to look. I had hints, of course. One old lady refused my offer of steroids for her Dachshund bitch and returned some months later claiming she had 'cured it with homeopathic sulphur'. I really didn't know what she was talking about. However, I was becoming aware that there was something else out there besides the limited number of conventional drugs upon which my medicine depended.

Being in an isolated area we were not in a position to refer patients for specialist treatment. My partner and I therefore became very skilful surgeons, and would happily embark on the most complex of orthopaedic reconstructions without a second thought. But I was becoming increasingly aware of the disparity between my surgical and medical success rates. And far too often I was viewing patients as cases, challenges to my intellect and skill, and often just as numbers in the waiting room to clear before I could get home. The satisfaction lay in solving the problem and gaining the respect of the client. Some way behind these goals came the physical welfare of my patients, and further behind again came their emotional welfare. This was the culmination of a process that had begun in veterinary school. With one or two exceptions, my tutors seemed to be motivated by ego and ambition rather than by a need to care for animals, and by the time I entered employment I had learnt the impersonality which most graduates show towards their patients, and often their clients. We were taught that to become emotionally involved with our patients would destroy us as veterinary surgeons as we would be unable to cope with the stress this would place on us. This process seems to have been further developed in the time since I qualified. An increasing reliance on laboratory tests ('work-ups') in the obsessive search for a diagnosis, and the associated jargon – all these serve to depersonalise the patient and allow the veterinary surgeon to see his patients as cases or case-loads rather than sentient beings with feelings and emotions. Gradually I became aware of this and in 1984 I went searching.

I was becoming increasingly interested in Eastern philosophy, I had briefly flirted with acupuncture, and needed a change. After six months wandering through south east Asia I returned to the UK for a while. Shortly after my return I saw an advertisement for an introductory day in veterinary homeopathy, run by veterinary surgeon Chris Day and Dr Jeremy Swaine, at Glastonbury. I found it fascinating. Chris had just published his book on the homoeopathic treatment of small animals (Day 1998). I bought a copy and read it from cover to cover. Shortly afterwards I started a locum appointment in Cardiff. I approached the principal about trying out homeopathy and to my eternal gratitude he agreed. My first serious homeopathic patient was an Old English Sheepdog who had been hit by a train some weeks beforehand. The vets in the practice had done a wonderful job of reconstructing his hindquarters but he had subsequently developed arthritis of the spine, to such an extent that he screamed with pain as soon as he tried to get up out of his bed. Once he was up and had moved a few paces he was fine but the pain of that first movement was dramatic. All the conventional anti-inflammatories and analgesics had helped for the first three or four days and had then lost their effect. Based on the modalities of 'worse for first movement, better for continued movement' I prescribed Rhus tox 6c twice daily. The result was truly miraculous: within a week all the pain had gone and at a follow-up consultation I was presented with a happy, energetic, freely moving dog – and a Parker pen! This was definitely something I needed to pursue.

Meanwhile, Big Ears had been released from quarantine with no sign of his allergy, but as soon as the spring came around he started scratching again. It took some months and several homeopathic medicines before I was able to control the itch, but happily he remained allergy-free for the remaining five years of his life. I finally ended his life to relieve him of the pain of cancer in 1989.

Over the next ten years I worked in nearly 30 practices, both in the UK and Australia, for periods ranging from one week to 18 months. In most of these practices I was able to develop my homeopathic prescribing skills and I was fortunate to spend several periods working for homeopathic vets such as Chris Day, John Saxton and Philippa Rodale, from all of whom I received valuable guidance and encouragement. I also attended the homeopathy courses at the London Homeopathic Hospital and qualified as a Vetinary Member of the Faculty of Homeopathy (VetMFHom) in 1991.

In 1995 I decided to branch out on my own and opened my own referral practice in Newcastle-Under-Lyme, Staffordshire, right next to the Peak District. I also used a colleague's branch practice in Grindleford, a small Derbyshire village not many miles from Dore. By this time Taz had come into my life, a Border Collie found wandering the streets of Poole. He was soon joined by Bunyip Bluegum Esq., a Jack Russell cross obtained from the rescue society close to Ashbourne in Derbyshire, where I lived. Taz taught me how to distinguish between Pulsatilla and Phosphorus in male dogs, a task which is not always as simple as it sounds; Bunyip developed a skin allergy and introduced me to the benefits of Tuberculinum for such patients.

In the course of my homeopathic education and studies, it became apparent that in order to make a homeopathic prescription on the deepest level, it was necessary to accept that animals are capable of experiencing feelings and emotions. In the *Organon*, Hahneman describes the overriding importance of mental changes in the patient as an expression of their disease, and his successors (Kent in particular) further emphasised this point. A cat who breaks out in miliary eczema after a new cat comes into the area, and who responds to Staphysagria (whose keynote is 'indignation') must surely be suffering from indignation and suppressed anger and I see no point in trying to argue to the contrary. Homeopathy has therefore brought me back to where I used to be, before modern veterinary training (almost) convinced me that our patients are subordinate beings who operate on a purely mechanistic level devoid of emotion, and that any projection of so-called human values onto such lower forms of life can be easily dismissed as 'anthropomorphism', a sin of the highest order!

Many of the patients presented to me for homeopathy in the Peak District were suffering from arthritis or an allied problem, and it came as an initial surprise to find how many of them seemed to respond to homeopathic Calc. fluor. I had used this remedy before, but never with the frequency with which I was prescribing it now. However, I soon realised it should not have been a surprise considering the prevalence of Calc. fluor, or fluorspar, in the Peak District. I had already been primed by Mark Elliot, working in West Sussex, who found he prescribed a disproportionate amount of Silica to horses with respiratory problems. The earth in that area, of course, is rich in flint, from which the homeopathic remedy silica is prepared. My childhood study of minerals had suddenly taken on a new meaning. The Doctrine of Signatures, to which the study of homeopathy had introduced me, suggests that the physical properties of a homeopathic remedy's source material give some indication of which patients may benefit from it. This helps to explain why I was presented with so many dogs whose radiographs of their limbs exhibit the typical 'crystalline' exostoses which are an indicator for the presciption of homeopathic Calc. fluor.

Since 2000 I have practised in East Sussex, a geologically diverse area among which can be found deposits of chalk and flint, clay and coal. I still prescribe Calc. fluor, but far more Calc. carb, Silica and particularly Graphites (pure carbon) than ever I used in the north. The study of homeopathy has brought me back to my childhood geological roots.

Many homeopathic remedies are made from plant material, and many of these, such as Hypericum perforatum and Bellis perennis, grow wild in the UK. Others are more exotic, while a large number were developed from Native American pharmacy. This being so, the last few years has rejuvenated my interest in our native flora. Most of the Bach flower remedies, while not strictly homeopathic but nevertheless developed by a homeo-path, are also developed from native British flowers and trees. The grounding that my mother gave me in identifying wild flowers has been the foundation for a study into the habits and appearance of plants on a far deeper level than simply 'putting a name to it'. Recently, Rajan Sankaran has published an analysis of the plant remedies used in homeopathy, classifying their symptomatologies according to their taxonomy (Sankaran 2002). This approach is not unique to him, and there are several other homeopaths working in the same area, but Sankaran has taken this concept forward to a degree well beyond anything heretofore. I have colleagues who have developed their interest in plant remedies with enormous enthusiasm, so much so that they have gone on to study herbal medicine; others have become attracted to the increasing number of flower remedies available, such as the Australian Bush Flower remedies developed by Ian White. So if flowers and plants are your interest, homeopathy can open new doors for you.

It was also in 1995 that I was approached by Chris Day and invited to become one of the core veterinary tutors on the veterinary course to commence with the Homeopathic Physicians Teaching Group (HPTG). I was unsure whether I had enough knowledge of homeopathy, but Chris assured me that enthusiasm was just as important! However, I had already delivered some lectures to the vets on the course at the Homeopathic Hospital and knew how much I enjoyed teaching. Furthermore it didn't take me long to realise that being a tutor at the HPTG would yield dividends beyond ego trips and fees; being a tutor with this group of individuals was going to be a journey of personal as well as academic growth. The founders of the HPTG were dynamic and disarmingly open, and they seemed to be operating on a level different from anything I was used to. Up to that point I had had no experience, and was probably quite sceptical, of any form of psychotherapy. To find that we had tutors' meetings under the supervision of a psychotherapeutic facilitator was a surprise, but I became increasingly aware of the value of such an approach, and indeed became more and more interested in this field. Later, I was introduced to the concept of supervision and of its value, and found our sessions with Robin Shohet immensely valuable, both professionally and personally. The processes that occur during supervision I find intriguing and immensely helpful when teaching generally, but especially in the supervision of tutorial groups, undergraduate and post-graduate. If one understands what happens in any situation where people (and animals) interact in a closed group it becomes clearer what are the real issues underlying the situation. For example, in one session I supervised, there were angry exchanges between some members of the group when we discussed the issue of the overvaccination of animals, and its consequences from a homeopathic point of view. Looking deeper revealed the anger which members of the group felt towards the vaccine companies for ignoring the problem.

Within a supervision group it is possible to tease out the real issues that are affecting the participants. Within a consultation, an understanding of the dynamics operating within the 'family' group of owners and animal can be of immense value in leading to a more skilful intervention than if only the more superficial information is used. For instance, an understanding of the emotional dynamics operating within a family, and the animal's role in this, can provide a deeper understanding of the disease process in operation. In supervision, role-play of the owner can reflect the dynamic as a parallel process to the consultation, and group dynamics can further enhance this understanding. This psychodynamic approach, both to homeopathic prescribing and to teaching, has opened up a whole new way of working for me, and indeed has given me a greater understanding of the actions and reactions of my clients, students and patients when faced with any particular situation. The concept of holism embodied in homeopathy is thus extended beyond the veterinary patient to the area of interaction with the extended family represented by owners and other animal companions.

Much of this psychodynamic approach to veterinary homeopathy comes as a result of the classes at the HPTG being of a mix of professions. Doctors and vets share most of the sessions, along with medical and sometimes veterinary nurses. Similarly, the class may be taught by a doctor or a vet or a team comprising one of each. The insights this provides for student and tutor alike facilitate the crosspollination of ideas that bears fruit during the process work that occurs in the supervision groups, particularly in the postgraduate course.

As an extension of these concepts, the interaction between remedy, patient and practitioner has, to me, become one of the most fascinating areas of research in medicine; there are phenomena at work here that defy the understanding of orthodox medicine. However, if we are to answer the criticisms of those who would prefer to ignore the evidence for homeopathy's effectiveness, then we have to at least attempt to find explanations for these phenomena. In considering the mechanism of potentisation of homeopathic remedies, I have been led to the work of those in the field of quantum physics, where the behaviour of sub-atomic particles defies many of the laws of Newton and is even influenced by the presence of an observer. Advances in the understanding of the physical laws which govern our universe demand a very different approach to the interpretation of experimental observations from that which we were taught at university. But there is no doubt in my mind that it is in this realm that explanations for the mechanism of action of homeopathy will be found. So if you are interested in quantum mechanics, chaos theory and similar fields, homeopathy can give you the opportunity to investigate them.

My HPTG colleagues have strongly influenced my thinking around the patient–owner–vet triad and hence it is my contention that such phenomena as transference and counter-transference, well accepted in the field of human psychology, are equally relevant to the veterinary consultation. It is important to understand that a client can transfer their issues and emotions onto the vet, and it is equally important to recognise that the vet can return the favour. So much of the skill of being a veterinary surgeon depends on developing an understanding of one's clients, as opposed to one's patients; it is they who must feel satisfied with the service they receive on behalf of their animal, otherwise they will not return and the veterinary surgeon's opportunity to aid the patient is lost.

The veterinary consultation represents an interaction on the same level as one within the medical context and an understanding of the processes that occur within it is of immense value if the prescriber is to make the maximum use of the time available. A large part of this is creating the atmosphere of trust that is vital to the continuing relationship between vet and client if the patient is to derive the benefit which homeopathy can provide. An understanding of psychodynamics facilitates this process. Increasingly, I find myself using the skills I am developing in supervision to gain a deeper understanding of the dynamics of disease in my patients. It is important to make sure that there is permission for this process, and as such the contract must be clear. However, it is only within a context of understanding that this contract can be made.

When it comes to the practicalities of making a homeopathic prescription it is the relationship between the owner and the patient that interests me most. Too often to be coincidence I find the owner of an animal has had the same remedy prescribed by a homeopath for themselves as that which I have just decided to give the dog or cat. Sometimes the owner and the patient are suffering from the same disease; at other times the symptoms are different but the two exhibit different facets of the same remedy. As a vet I also come across clients who have had more than one, and often a series, of pets suffering from the same disease.

So what is it that produces these effects? We know that people often select dogs or cats that resemble them physically, but the phenomenon I am describing must surely operate at a deeper level. My own peripatetic lifestyle is typical of someone with a deeply entrenched tubercular miasm, but Bunyip didn't necessarily know this when he exhibited signs of the remedy Tuberculinum. In fact he also needed a follow-up prescription of Rhus tox to complete the cure, but perhaps this is a hint to me to take my stiff back more seriously. He has also exhibited signs of natrum muriaticum when I was myself undergoing a grieving process. Taz on the other hand broke out in a rash at the same time as I needed Pulsatilla for prostate pain. I observe this sort of correlation so often that I now usually seek permission to investigate some of my clients' issues in life when prescribing for their animals. The majority of my clients are quite ready to accept that the correlation exists and to co-operate in this process. If they are reluctant to do so, then that gives me similarly useful information.

My experience is that accepting that this phenomenon exists means it can be put to use in filling some of the gaps that the veterinary homeopathic consultation normally leaves. Just as in medical homeopathy, it is essential to incorporate an assessment of the patient's mental and emotional state in the symptom picture. However, it has to be accepted that in the case of an animal, this is not the description of the patient; rather it is a subjective interpretation by the vet and the owner of the animal's behaviour. Accepting the close relationship between the owner and the animal as I have described renders symptoms on the mental and emotional plane more accessible – indeed, they may be more readily understood if expressed by the owner personally rather than guessed at from the behaviour of the animal. Put simply, it is my contention that if the emotional state, as deduced from an interpretation of the animal's behaviour, is mirrored in the owner then it is more reliable. There are of course numerous pitfalls in this approach, but my experience is that it can be a valuable tool.

Why these phenomena of correspondence should be so I do not know, but I am brave enough to suggest that there may be some agreement on a higher level that the pet will reflect the needs of its 'owner'. Here I have inserted inverted commas as it is at this point that the concept of owner and pet ceases to be appropriate. What other epithet one chooses I leave to the reader, but considering such a connection between animal and human places the animal beyond the position it occupies in Western society, and affords it a respect more in accordance with that of the Eastern philosophies such as Hinduism and Buddhism. I see this as not only positive for the animal, but also for the observer, for it demands compassion.

The foregoing may well engender feelings and emotions in the reader, and perhaps the most important point in this discussion is the observation that from my early investigations into a way of treating allergic skin disease more effectively, homeopathy has led me into the realms of metaphysics, as well as physics. It is this that enthuses me about homeopathy: wherever your interest lies, homeopathy has the ability to satisfy the need. If you are interested in plants it can take you into the study of taxonomy, of toxicology and of horticulture. If you are interested in chemistry you can study the periodic table and develop its use following the work of Scholten (1996). If you are interested in philosophy and psychology, homeopathy can lead you into areas of self-development hitherto hidden to you. If physics is your stuff then grapple with the phenomena of potentisation and remedy reactions.

For myself, homeopathy has brought me into a realm of experience with a breadth and depth that at one time I could not have imagined. My professional consultations are often a treasure trove of discovery, as I observe the exchanges of energy between my client and patient and try to interpret my own feelings. That is on a good day. On a bad day I can only see the obvious, the surface of the process; sometimes even that is obscured and I convince myself that I am unworthy to call myself 'homeopath' never mind 'tutor'. It is important to experience this, as it is part of my duty as tutor to support my students in their journey of self-discovery. If I can still feel what they feel I am better placed to offer support. Similarly, I still make mistakes, and that's alright too, as I need to be able to help my students see their 'mistakes' as seriously useful opportunities to learn.

More than ever I listen to my patients and try to understand them, I listen to my clients and try to understand them, and I listen to my dog and I try to work out what he is trying to tell me. I listen to myself and try to understand me, and with the skills I have learned through studying homeopathy, and even more so through teaching with the HPTG I am beginning to make sense. The examples, wisdom and support of my fellow tutors have been of immense value in this. As we strive to deal with the issues which inevitably surface in the running of the HPTG and those which inevitably surface from working together, we put into practice what we have learnt from our supervisors, and from each other, and we continually strive to develop our teaching skills in the same manner.

For the last few years I have had the privilege of teaching homeopathy in foreign countries, mainly under the auspices of HPTG International, but also independently. This satisfies my passion for travel, and gives me that satisfaction of sharing what I have learned with a wider audience. The same changes in perception which I observe occurring as students progress through the Oxford course I recognise in our students in Australia and Ireland, and it is a joy to see how people's lives change positively as a result. Providing the support as these changes occur is an essential responsibility for the HPTG, and my own process work within the organisation renders me better equipped to fulfil that role.

All in all, practising and teaching homeopathy has taken me on a journey of self-discovery that has enriched my life inestimably. It is this journey that I endeavour to share with all those beings I encounter in my life, professional or otherwise. As sentient beings we live in a complex world of processes that operate on a level beyond that within which we normally function. Homeopathy reflects this complexity and helps us to become aware of some of the phenomena that represent the workings of our universe. This is a long way from treating a dog's arthritis with Rhus tox; such is the journey upon which we embark when we choose to investigate homeopathy.

References

Day, C. (1998) *Homoeopathic Treatment of Small Animals: Principles and Practice* 3rd edition. London: E.W. Daniel Co. Ltd.

Hahnemann, S. (1982) *Organon of Medicine.* 5th and 6th edition. New Delhi: B. Jain Publishers. Translated by R.E. Dudgeon.

Kent, J.J. (1995) *Lectures on Homoeopathic Philosophy.* New Delhi: B. Jain Publishers.

Sankaran, R. (2002) *An Insight into Plants.* Mumbai: Homeopathic Medical Publishers.

Scholten, J. (1996) *Homeopathy and the Elements.* Utrecht: Stichting Alonnissos.

Introduction to Chapter 5

John Saxton's chapter is, in many ways, quite different from the others. His journey has taken him from the blind acceptance of conventional medicine to a realisation, based on his clinical empiricial evidence with animals, that homeopathy was a very effective alternative – not what he would have expected given his early background. John does not give us as many autobiographical details as the other writers, seeing it perhaps as self-indulgent to be writing too much in the first person. Nevertheless, he shares his passion when describing the dangers he sees when conventional medicine is too reliant on science at the expense of paying attention to nature.

When I asked John what was the most important message he wanted readers to take from reading his piece, he replied:

> It is important for people to realise that, in the final analysis, they are responsible for their own health and where appropriate, for that of the animals in their care. It must also be remembered that the body, be it human or animal, is designed to be healthy and to restore itself to health when sick. Good health is nature's natural state of affairs, not a reward for good behaviour to be awarded by the medical or veterinary profession. All treatments and procedures should first be judged against the basic criterion of 'Does this work with or against nature?' before other factors are considered.

Chapter 5

The Betrayal of Nature
John Saxton

A drug is a chemical which, when injected into a laboratory animal, will produce a scientific paper.

Professor William Paton

The foundation

Some years ago, during one of the regular flu warnings that are issued at the beginning of most British autumns, a doctor, being interviewed on television about the illness and its threat, made a highly significant remark. One which, in fact, could be classed almost as a Freudian slip. On being asked by the interviewer what could be done about the condition, his reply was that 'There is no known cure; *all* we can do is to let nature take its course.'

I have added the italics because it seems to me that they illustrate the thought process and attitude behind the doctor's words. It is an attitude that, albeit subconsciously, appears to run through much of modern medical thought and, when taken to extremes, leads to as many problems as it solves. In the event, the advice that the doctor gave was in the main eminently sensible, namely rest, fluids and time while the body did its own curative work. But to me the implication that he regarded this as second best to what modern medicine ought to be able to achieve was unmistakable.

However, there was a time when I would have accepted, indeed welcomed, such an assertion of medicine's healing superiority, and poured scorn on any suggestion that nature could ever do better on its own than it could with the help of modern science. Any other view at that time would have been heresy!

My training had been based on science, but behind the detail there was another idea being sown and taking root. That was that science, rather than being just a means of explaining and helping nature had, in a way, become superior to it, and could be used to improve on and exploit what the natural order had created. Forty years ago that was, for many of us, a very seductive philosophy. There was no doubt then that the age of modern medicine had arrived, and the benefits of drugs such as antibiotics were being widely felt and welcomed. New equipment for improved surgical and investigative techniques was appearing in a steady stream of innovation. For me, a generally conventionally minded individual, coming from a background closely allied to, but not directly involved with, conventional medical practice, all this appeared natural, in a way inevitable, and certainly desirable.

Why did I choose any medical discipline as a career, and why become a vet and not a doctor? It was certainly no coldly reasoned decision, and the only accurate answer is that it seemed to me to be 'a good idea at the time' – and that time was early. I moved straight from the standard boyhood dream of wanting to be an engine driver to planning to be a vet, and for some reason the human medical profession was never seriously considered. I was certainly no Francis of Assisi in disguise, and had no feeling of a desperate need to heal individual animals. Looking back, it may be that it was another aspect of my receptivity to the scientific approach, thinking in terms of numbers rather than individuals. But yet at the same time, there was never any question of a career in research; clinical practice was always the aim. There may also have been an element of pragmatic cowardice in there as well, with a subconscious feeling that although it didn't really matter if one killed a few animals by mistake, generally it was not considered a good thing to kill too many people!

My time at college provided me with two major strands of influence. From the formal tuition came the extolling of new scientific developments, and the widening of opportunities that these presented. From my contacts with vets out in practice, many of whom had worked during the pre-chemical revolution (prior to the advent of chemically-orientated drugs), came a confirmatory welcoming of the new therapeutic agents, and an enthusiasm for the new powers that were being added to their armoury. And so, in the fullness of time, I and the others in my generation of new graduates entered the profession, feeling that we were being provided with the best of all worlds. We had been exposed to the methods and philosophy of the older practitioners, and could take much from that, whilst science would provide any tool that we needed to help our endeavours. For me there was initially no question of practising in any other way than the strictly conventional, and for some 15 years that was the course I followed. There were unfortunately some clinical failures. However, some failures were regarded as an inevitable and permanent feature of medical life, and whilst we were encouraged to question the application of the method in these cases, there was never any question of doubting the method itself.

And so, from this start, how did I end up being classed (wrongly) as a rebel and writing a chapter in a book like this? Why do I feel that in many ways I have more in common with people such as my co-authors of this book, than I do with many of my conventional colleagues? Where along the way did orthodox medicine lose both the plot and me? The process of my conversion is the story of my reaction to what I have perceived as the errors and limitations of modern medicine.

Broadening the perspective

For me, the major error that has developed within the conventional system has been the increasingly narrow scientific nature of medical training, and the growing conviction that science could provide all the answers, not only to the existing problems, but also to questions that had not yet been dreamt of, let alone asked. And as new questions were thought of, and as the medical generations passed, the training of all disciplines became more scientifically orientated. New doctors and vets were being indoctrinated with the power of science rather than the power of nature, and it became more and more the function of medical science to provide what the professions and the public wanted rather than solely what they needed.

Over the years it became apparent to me that, increasingly, what both the medical and veterinary professions wanted was to be able to control and direct nature. In fairness, much of the drive for this originated from society in general, which had been led to believe that science could do almost anything for them, but it resonated with the new ultra-scientific ethos of the medical world. The worthy aims of the relief of suffering and the prevention of illness, which had always been there, became expanded into the concept that nothing and no one must ever be allowed to experience the slightest pain or discomfort, nothing or no one must ever be allowed to become ill, and no one must be inconvenienced by the constraints of biology and nature's rules, if some chemical agent or surgical procedure could possibly be found to avoid it.

As science was increasingly seen as the means of achieving these goals, so the ways of science were presented as the golden pathway to the Promised Land. For me, however, the interpretation and application of the scientific method that I saw became increasingly narrow. Scientific research is, of course, dependent in every situation on having something that is measurable. However, the degree of standardisation that is now being applied before it is considered that any valid conclusions can be drawn appears to be restrictive. The approach is a useful tool up to a point, and its use has added much that is valuable to medical knowledge and practice, but when it is taken to extremes as the only method of investigation, it seems to be blocking rather than enhancing progress. With the passage of time the body has come to be regarded merely as an entity consisting of large numbers of small measurable units, to be analysed, separated and put back together in a slightly different pattern that better suited the dictates of control than the original. And thus the individual patient has become just another physical unit to be fitted into a scientific straitjacket.

Whether my introduction to homoeopathy is regarded as coincidence, serendipity, or divine intervention, the fact remains that it occurred at such a time and in such a way that it did not seem to pose a threat to my existing beliefs and practices. A notice of a meeting organised by the British Homeopathic Association, 'A Veterinary Seminar on Homeopathy', for some reason caught my eye. For some equally unknown reason I decided to attend, and found four experienced veterinary surgeons expounding the virtues of homoeopathy, and doing so from the point of view of proven clinical practice, not abstract theory. This was a refreshing change from the approach to which I was being constantly subjected by drug firms and other professional colleagues. Here, it appeared, was a new range of therapeutic options that could be used alongside the proven methods of established medicine. However, while I did not appreciate the full implications of the new methods at the time, it soon became clear to me that not only could the new agents equal the performance of the existing therapeutics, but they could in certain circumstances exceed them. It was one thing to find that homoeopathic remedies such as Aconite and Arnica gave better results in the acute treatment of victims of road traffic incidents than steroids did, but the realisation that in other cases different remedies produced more satisfactory results than their 'conventional equivalents' gave food for thought.

The reason for this was that I was basing my assessment solely on what I saw before my eyes in the surgery. For me the sole objective of practice was to cure patients, and anything that achieved that was acceptable. And the best curative agents, no matter what they were or where they came from, were the most acceptable. Even before any recognised change in my methods occurred, already I was basing my approach to medicine on the opening exhortation of the basic philosophical work of homoeopathy, the *Organon*, namely that 'The physician's highest and only calling is to make the sick healthy'. There was, it is true, still some confusion in my mind between the removal of symptoms and genuine cure, but that would change with time.

All this was, of course, in contrast to the increasingly 'evidenced-based direction' that the establishment was moving towards. The idea that 'if science can't prove it then it can't work' became for me increasingly at odds with the obvious facts of clinical life as I saw them. The mere use of different types of medicines gave way to a realisation that these agents were linked to a different philosophy of medicine. I began to question, tentatively at first, the whole basis of the conventional scientific approach as applied to medicine.

It was a process that took many years. At first, perhaps inevitably, I attempted to fit homoeopathy into the pattern of conventional medicine as I knew it. This course led me into a blind alley, and I came to realise that beyond a certain point medicine and a narrow view of science are incompatible. When I thought about my scientific training I realised that the pure scientific approach is that of the pessimist. The main approach to any theory that is proposed is to test it by trying to disprove it. It is only when that process has failed that the theory is accepted as valid. In their private lives, individual scientists may be the greatest of extroverts and optimists, but professionally their approach is pessimistic and sceptical. True clinicians, in contrast, are professional optimists, always hoping for, searching for and expecting a cure. The real clinician would never accept the premise that 'it hasn't been proved to work, therefore it must not be tried'. That is the realm of the medical or veterinary scientist who happens to be in clinical practice. And such a scientist also falls within the definition of 'someone who cannot see something working in practice without asking whether it would work in theory' – a definite case of inverted priorities!

For true clinicians the only valid consideration is a patient who is cured and who remains cured. Those of us who accept this recognise an increasing gulf opening between ourselves and our colleagues. Those who require the independent validation of a 'science' before they will trust either their own judgement or accept their own results can become prey to doubts and frustrations, and ultimately these feelings may filter through to their patients and clients, to the detriment of all. The doubts and frustrations of these practitioners are compounded by the fact that they limit their interpretation of the scientific method to a very narrow perspective. Half their time is spent stuck in the time warp of Newtonian physics, and the other half worshipping the sacred cow of what is, for them, the only acceptable measure of efficiency: the controlled and randomised 'double blind trial'.

I came to realise that those who insist that homoeopathy must fit into the established patterns of so-called scientific medicine limit both themselves and their patients. For some, their 'scientific' view precludes serious consideration of any therapy other than the conventional. Others use homoeopathic remedies, as I did initially, because the remedies are seen to work to a level, albeit superficial. But because they are not prepared, due to the constraints of their view of science, to take that leap into an understanding of why remedies work, they can never appreciate the true potential of the homoeopathic healing method, or indeed the true potential of healing itself. In essence they regard remedies as just another group of medicines, to be used in the same way as any other group.

In the final analysis, their criterion of acceptability is someone else's approval and validation. This means that they never come to appreciate exactly what is happening in the body during illness and that is their, and medicine's, ultimate tragedy. Their failure to move beyond the confines of their so-called scientific view of medicine means that, even if they use homoeopathic remedies at a superficial level, the whole philosophy by which they work is in fact, at its roots, indistinguishable from that which governs the thought processes of their totally conventional professional colleagues. All of these, via their science, may be able to explain how the body functions, but not the ultimate why. And as a consequence they fail to appreciate that the ability to change a physiological process is not necessarily the same as the desirability of doing so. Such a philosophy has science increasingly at its centre with nature at the periphery, as opposed to the true healing philosophy that has nature at its centre, with science as an obedient acolyte.

Once nature has been removed from the central position, then the idea of universal freedom from pain or inconvenience becomes, in theory, a realisable goal. In practice, however, we know that it doesn't work out like that. Francis Bacon (1620) said that 'nature cannot be ordered about, except by obeying her'. If nature is ignored or abused she has a habit of fighting back. Unfortunately, the conventional response to that fightback is often simply not to realise why it is happening, and to attempt to impose further controls. Once I had accepted this, the next stage was easy. It was the realisation that nature had to be put back at the centre of the clinical process if true healing was to be achieved.

I had become part of a profession which, along with our medical colleagues, had been fighting disease for hundreds of years. But nature, I knew, has been doing so for millions, evolving and adapting as she went along in order to develop the perfect system. And the fact of the survival and development of life on earth was testament to her success. And yet increasingly among many of my colleagues there appeared to be a reluctance to take account of that: an unwillingness to look at any situation from the starting point of 'How does nature deal with this problem?'

This reluctance stemmed in part from the way in which medicine had developed historically. The influence of Galen, the Greek physician who first defined the individual organs of the body, and others since his time, has developed into the reductionist approach to healing, which is very much in accord with the scientific ethos of 'Break it down into isolated and measurable parts, and then measure everything in sight'. This drive towards what is effectively an oversimplification has resulted in the development of germ theory, with its 'cause and effect' thinking, which is, in many ways, an oversimplification. Another loss along the way has been the separation of the material and spiritual aspects of life. This has resulted in the idea that the whole is merely the sum of the parts, rather than the truly holistic concept that the whole is more than just the combined effect of individual systems.

Another result has been what could be called the triumph of immediate measurable results over the search for deep significant change, and this has led to the confusion between mere removal of symptoms and genuine cure. The symptoms have come to be regarded as the disease merely because they are finite, and the logical step from that is to regard the removal of symptoms as synonymous with cure.

Most of my attempts to discuss these ideas with colleagues were met not only with a failure to understand, but with an unwillingness even to try to understand. Their belief system apparently took little account of any realities outside its own certainties. Fortunately, there were others whom I met, first within the veterinary profession, and then additionally among the doctors, who also realised that the disease process was the vital element, and that that alone was the key to understanding and cure. As a result we all acknowledged the need to approach healing from a broader perspective, to break free from what we saw as the dominating and ultimately deadening hand of a very narrow view of science, and to view everything once more from the purely clinical and functional aspect.

The deficiencies exposed

Once I begin to measure the modern developments and attitudes of scientific medicine against this basic fact of healing, it quickly becomes apparent to me how far things have gone astray. First, in the curative situation, the overriding concentration on the removal of symptoms and lesions, together with the obsession that all discomfort, let alone suffering, must be removed at all cost, has led to the application of therapeutic measures that oppose rather than assist nature. Anti-pyretic agents, to artificially reduce fever, and anti-inflammatory drugs to fulfil a similar function, are used extensively to counter bodily processes and symptoms, without any regard as to why those processes are occurring in the first place. Conventionally, they are not seen as positive guides to the natural mechanisms of cure, but are regarded as the undesirable developments of disease, to be removed or suppressed above any other consideration. And the mere removal of symptoms is increasingly being equated with cure. Analgesia has also become an obsession, to be achieved at all costs, even at the price of interfering with an ongoing healing process. Although much analgesia is not only ethically but medically desirable, it is being taken to extremes. There is in fact a big difference between 'unnecessary suffering' and 'necessary discomfort', but often this is a distinction that seems either not to be appreciated or to be ignored by my conventional colleagues. It appears that medicine is, in many cases, forcing nature to fight disease with one hand tied behind her back. The working through of natural processes is a prerequisite of true healing, and many conventional practices are appearing increasingly counterproductive.

And yet I felt that there was obviously still much of value in what the conventional scientific approach had created, and patients were served best by utilising those parts within a broader concept of healing, while rejecting the rest. And surely I could expect many of those best parts to be found in the field of preventive medicine? Even though the treatment of disease seemed in many ways to be moving along the wrong lines, if disease could be prevented, that was the ultimate aim, and had the advantage that it would avoid the later pitfalls of wrongly directed treatment. Of course, much had been achieved already in this direction. Improvements in diet and hygiene had yielded immense benefits. And then there was the miracle of vaccination!

At least that was how, by inference, it was presented to us at college. Looking back, I realised that we had been taught very little about vaccination in our initial training, and yet the ethos had been established that vaccination was undoubtedly a good thing, and that it was a clinical course that should be followed at every possible opportunity. And this ethos had grown during my early years in practice, as new vaccines were developed for an increasing range of conditions. It had become the ultimate expression of the idea that 'nothing and nobody must be allowed to become ill if it can be avoided'.

But that realisation has reinforced the concerns that were beginning to surface when it became clear to me that, in the pursuit of this objective, science itself has suspended the critical faculty that it applies to all else. Again, as in other situations, it was the lodestar of clinical observation that revealed the first doubts; there were just too many clinical situations involving illness following vaccination for it to be coincidence. But the vehemence that greeted any criticism of vaccination was far greater than in any other situation. It has become apparent to me that all discussions and investigations start from the article of faith that vaccinations are without doubt safe except for, proportionally, a very few cases. Even in these cases there appears to be an implication that the fault lies with the individual rather than the vaccine, and certainly not with the principle of vaccination. While it was undoubtedly true that the 'headline tragedies' associated with vaccination were mercifully few compared to the doses administered, equally it was becoming clear to many of us that a lot of lesser but nonetheless serious consequences could be laid at the procedure's door.

Vaccination, of course, has done much good. But the open-minded can see that it is also doing harm that is not being acknowledged. The philosophy and techniques of modern vaccination have developed away from the original concepts and methods. Both the agents used and the means of administration have been developed from the point of view of scientific theory, and the one question that has not been asked along the way is why nature has done things in the way that she has. The massive amounts of information that have been accumulated over the years show in mind-boggling detail how the immune system functions, but that only answers the 'how' and not the 'why'. Again, I consider that nature has been removed from the heart of the process.

It also appears to many of us that the tool of science, which has led to this situation, is in some ways being used to maintain it, and to block any serious re-appraisal of the situation. All that is needed is an honest look at the issues in a spirit of truly scientific enquiry. It is accepted that all the other groups of powerful agents used in medicine are capable of producing profound effects for both good and ill. Surely it defies logic that vaccines should be the exception? From this point, surely it is an obvious clinical step to consider the possibility of side effects and acknowledge them when they are found?

There are many of us who are in no doubt that untoward effects are being seen as a result of vaccination. But those of us who are finding them are, at best, being ignored, or at worst, vilified, for thinking what science has decreed to be the unthinkable. After all, our ideas have only come from the field of clinical experience and observation of nature rather than from the more reliable cold, dispassionate realm of the 'God of Science'!

To those of us who have come to realise that there is a better way of healing, one that obeys the basic rule of assisting rather than attempting to dominate nature, all of these developments are to varying degrees both worrying and depressing. However, it appears to us that we are now facing a situation where medical science is following an even more dangerous course, one that manifests its own controlling instincts in an entirely new way. It is moving from attempting to dominate nature to trying to defy it. For many of us this is a frightening development, not only from the point of view of individual health, but also for what it implies in relation to the future development of medicine.

It is well known that for centuries mankind has attempted to influence the requirements and physiology of reproduction. All kinds of religious and social influences have come into play in this regard, but medicine has been essentially powerless to make any major contribution. Hence the emphasis has until recently been on what might be termed 'mechanical' measures. Modern advances in physiological understanding now mean that at last medicine can intervene. Whether it is wise to do so has been a question that has not been given much consideration. It is true that much discussion has taken place from the human socio-ethical point of view, but not so much from the purely medical. The possible effects on the health of the individual have not been given as high a priority as they deserved, because control, not health, has been the driving force. An increasing number of us believe that although up to now science in medicine has at least been attempting always to heal, that is now being left behind. A 'brave new world' of medicine has begun which has entered the field of social engineering.

Both increasing and decreasing reproductive activity offer opportunities for manipulation. In agriculture, efforts have always been made to manage reproduction, but the old means have been essentially natural, via timing of matings, etc. Indeed, many of the older management systems were devised because of the reproductive limitations imposed by nature. However, all that has changed. The female reproductive cycle can now be controlled and altered by chemical means, to fit in with purely economic requirements. And if these new methods happen to give rise to individual health problems, that is of no consequence as the results can be, if not buried, at least eaten. Such reservations as are voiced concern the effects on human health rather than on the health of the animals involved.

In human medicine, although the approach is more individually based, the aim is essentially the same: control. And the means employed, in treatments such as in vitro fertilization, use chemical agents to control and alter the natural situation at the whim of individuals, often for social rather than medical reasons.

At first glance it is easy to think that to increase the reproductive capacity of either a species or an individual is entirely in accord with nature, as reproduction is so vital to the survival of a species, nature's priority. However, problems can arise because of the way it is done, namely by means of altering the natural cycles and processes using chemical means. But it is at the other end of the reproductive spectrum that some of us are finding the worst abuses, where there is a direct clash with natural function, and where the aim of the interference is either to suppress reproductive activity or (additionally in humans) to prolong it beyond its normal limits.

Surgical neutering of animals has both social and medical justifications, but it appears obvious to us that continuously to suppress the reproductive cyclic activity in an entire female of any species by chemical means can cause many more serious problems. The presence of a reproductive system that is trying to function normally in accord with nature, and whose outlets are being blocked constantly, can result in the system turning in on itself and producing major and dangerous disease.

Essentially we see the same situation at the other end of human reproductive life with the menopause. Here also medicine and science have attempted to solve the undoubted problems associated with it by refusing to consider and co-operate with nature. There is no consideration of why the menopause exists as a natural phenomenon. We know that nature does not do anything for the sake of it, and so the menopause must have a positive function. But the conventional approach is to attempt to abolish it by extending the previous sexually active phase of life, the very thing that nature is trying to draw to a close. Again, it is another form of interference with a tried and tested system that leads inevitably to problems.

That these 'social manipulations' are causing many clinical problems is well recognised by those who are dealing with the consequences. Mammary and cervical malignancies following chemical suppression are not uncommon, upsets to normal fertility occur, and other uterine conditions requiring radical treatment are regular elements of the daily case-load, as well as more widespread upsets affecting other areas of the body.

Facing the consequences

It is obvious to all that the major health problems of the present day are no longer the major epidemics of the past. What is now being seen is a steady increase in chronic diseases of all sorts, and the emergence of new acute infections. The incidence of cancer, arthritis, asthma, etc. is rising in spite of the vast and increasing range of options available to the modern clinician. When we look at the numbers involved, many of us feel that we are in an epidemic of chronic disease that makes the Black Death seem like a minor inconvenience! And every new medical development appears either to create new problems, or at best change the nature of the old ones. Mankind has been warned that nature will always bite back, and now it seems that we are seeing just that with increasing frequency, as the level of interference rises.

For those who wish to see change, this does not involve the renunciation of science, but rather the realisation that in the final analysis there is no such thing as the 'science of healing'. The proponents of the 'scientific' method deride the empirical as unsound, and yet essentially the empirical is neither more nor less than the utilisation of experience. And yet how sound is a method that discounts the ultimate proof that is clinical experience in favour of a theoretical basis backed by standardisation, testing formats sanitised from real-life situations and the ultimate denial of the individual? A true understanding of nature's processes is more important than any number of isolated trials, especially when these are conducted without due regard for nature's criteria.

Those who have put nature back once more where she belongs are not saying that science has nothing to offer healing. It has much to contribute, but it is as a servant not as a master. The straitjacket that modern medicine has created by its selective use of scientific thinking is, in my opinion, both stifling the development of medicine, and also leading it in the wrong direction. True science is nothing more or less than the pursuit of knowledge in all forms. As my colleague and co-author, Peter Gregory, wrote in the Veterinary Times (2003, pp.3–4):

> The (true) scientific method is the triad of observation, hypothesis and experiment which serves to add to the body of knowledge. We can safely assume that it was this method which primitive man employed when rubbing two sticks together to make fire. It is uncertain how many placebo-

controlled randomised trials were performed before the principle was accepted.

For me the change towards a narrow view of science in the approach of medicine over my working life has been profound. Science has come to dominate not only its methodology but also its technology and its morality. The old and honourable concept of simply curing is now being limited to 'curing by scientific means' with scientifically measurable criteria of 'cure' and maximum use being made of sophisticated 'toys', often seemingly merely because they exist. The equally honourable concept of disease prevention is now increasingly either a question of screening programmes (which fail to ask why the disease exists at all) or vaccination on the most massive scale possible without even considering the possibility of significant detrimental effects. A health service is generally hailed as a success if it treats increasing numbers of patients, but in fact a truly successful health service would need to be treating less patients year by year.

And now science, having led medicine away from attempting to work with nature to achieve its ends, has gone the whole way and is now openly attempting to defy nature – definitely a concept too far! Hence we now have cloning, test-tube babies, foetal sex selection and the prospect of the triumph of the 'science is God' mentality.

Medicine may appear to be helping more and more people with more and more problems, and the views expressed in this chapter will be countered by many with examples of the progress that has been made. However, it seems to many of us that this progress is being bought at a high price, and that there is an increasing betrayal of both those that medicine purports to help, and those that enter the healing professions with a genuine desire to cure. It is this trend that we at the Homeopathic Professionals Teaching Group (HPTG) wish to reverse.

We are a group of very different individuals, with different perspectives, but with a common purpose: to raise awareness of healing's true potential.

It is not a question of repudiating all that has gone before, but of placing it in its true context and using all the available methods to heal, with an open mind and a genuine spirit of enquiry.

The parallel with one of the major developments in homoeopathy is fascinating. Many of Hahnemann's early followers thought that all that was needed to cure all disease was more and more remedies, and a better understanding of them. Hahnemann, however, thought that this was too simplistic a view, and by going back and considering nature's way of responding to disease, he was able to make his great leap forward in his understanding of chronic disease. Today we have science telling us that all that is needed is more science, more medicines, more techniques and all disease will be eliminated. What is really needed is another great leap back to, and willingness to learn from, nature.

References

Gregory, P. (2003) *Veterinary Times,* 4 August 2003.

Hahnemann, S. (1982) *Organon of Medicine.* 5th & 6th edition. New Dehli: B. Jain Publishers. Translated by. R.E. Dudgeon.

Introduction to Chapter 6

David Curtin's journey, like those of the other authors, has taken him out of conventional and into complementary medicine. What is particularly interesting is that at the time of writing he has just gone back into conventional medicine and is enjoying it. Given all the alternatives he has tried, it shows that the two forms of medicine can be integrated. David writes, 'Every case is an opportunity for the doctor to bring his or her passion for life into the consulting room and perhaps to help the patient to discover their own.' I would love a sequel to this chapter describing his work in the NHS.

When I asked David what was the most important message he would like the reader to take away from his writing he replied:

> Health and sickness appear to be opposites, but like a glass that may be either half empty or half full, depending on how you view it, a person's attitude to his or her health can radically affect how his sickness or health affects his or her life. A true physician can facilitate a person in effecting the changes that may be curative.

Chapter 6

Discovering the Art of Healing – A Doctor's Journey
David Curtin

Early influences

I had wanted to be a doctor for as long as I could remember. There was no history of medicine in the family nor did I know any doctors, so I don't really know where the idea came from. I wanted to know how everything worked – how electricity worked, how cars worked, how the body worked. I didn't care about people particularly, not in the caring, sympathetic sense. Medicine for me was about science. It was also about fixing people, healing their hurts; maybe I liked the power. I was certainly attracted to the status that being a doctor carried, and the possibility of a good income. I think that the relatively poor background from which my father had come was a stimulus. He was raised as a strict Roman Catholic and remained so all his life. He never achieved the success that he really wanted. He struggled with life, lacked confidence and did not socialise easily, but he was a most remarkable man. He was extraordinarily conscientious, profoundly moral and totally dedicated to his family. He did very little for himself. Though I rebelled against what I perceived as his authoritarianism, I have no doubt that he had a great influence on me, and probably I am very much like him. I can remember being shocked on my first visit to Ireland and my father's childhood home at the age of three. As we got off the ferry at Cork there were men and boys running around in bare feet, offering to carry our bags for a few coppers. I was also amazed at the single cold tap in the yard at my grandmother's house, and the outside toilet with the sheets of newspaper. And of course there was the pig in its sty just over the wall and the smell that went with it, and the potato patch instead of a lawn. When I think of it now I remember the wonderfully fresh air, and the majestic view sweeping from the back yard right up to the 3000-foot peak of Galtymore a dozen miles away.

Medical school

I never had any doubts about getting into medical school. I did take a year off before I started, nowadays called a gap year, and taught chemistry at residential sixth form college in Nairobi. I wanted adventure, and Africa seemed like a great place to go and get it. One of my duties was driving the students around in the college van, to football matches and various other engagements with other schools. I got to see a lot of east Africa as a result. One of the trips was to a science fair in Dar es Salaam. We went overland through Masai country, and very close to the foot of Mount Kilimanjaro. I shall never forget my first view of that snow-capped crater seemingly hanging there in the sky in the early evening. I also went on an expedition collecting plant specimens on Mount Kenya with the biology teacher and some of his students. The plants were for a research project run by an Italian university. I have had a taste for travel and adventure ever since. The first two years at Guy's Hospital were packed with factual learning – too much. My brain rebelled against it and I really had to force myself to study. Much of the detail we had to learn seemed to me to be irrelevant. Useful no doubt, for specialist surgeons or biochemists, but not for the general doctor. For the first time in my life I considered the possibility that I might fail an examination. Fortunately I passed and went on to the next stage: three years of ward work. I didn't enjoy it at all. Consultant ward rounds were conducted like military parades. The team would line up outside the ward awaiting the great man's arrival (and the great men were all men). When he arrived, the procession would proceed in order of consultant, ward sister, junior medical staff, staff nurses and finally medical students. The patients would be discussed and sometimes interrogated, the medical students grilled, and finally pro-nouncements would be made. The junior doctors would go round later to explain to the patients what had happened. I was already becoming a bit of rebel. Strict hierarchies and mili-tarism were not my style.

Many patients did not respond to treatment, and I rapidly became disillusioned. I think I had assumed that modern medicine had all the answers and that most diseases could fairly easily be cured. It was a bit of a shock to find that this was not the case – perhaps I was was more naïve than most. I might have dropped out, but I had always been so single-mindedly determined to be a doctor that to do so was virtually impossible for me.

Discovering meditation

At the same time I was becoming very interested in the esoteric, reading the works of Gurdjieff, Ouspensky and many others. The philosophy of the Indian yogis interested me particularly and I began meditating regularly, initially the kriya yoga and then other techniques. This and my teacher were to have a profound effect on my life. I developed a sense of inner peace and joy. I think that it had always been there, but it became clearer and more accessible. That is not to say that I did not have worries, fears, moments of sadness, anger, frustration, and all the other emotions that are part of being a human being. But these seemed transitory and superficial in comparison. The sense of inner joy has never really left me since, even though I have been irregular in my meditation in recent years. I do notice, though, that when I do meditate I am always closer to my centre.

I had always taken it for granted that things would go well for me in life, and generally they did. My father called it 'David's luck'. If I went on holiday the sun always shone. If I wanted a job, or whatever it was, I always seemed to get it. Luck may have indeed played a part, but I know that I always looked on the bright side, and those things that didn't go well I quickly forgot. I think I probably inherited this from my mother who has always been an extremely positive person. I have never known anything get her down for long. She will always find a reason to celebrate the joy of being alive.

Discovering homeopathy

While in my final year at medical school, I was introduced to homeopathy by a fellow medical student. He took me to some lectures at the Royal London Homoeopathic Hospital (RLHH). I was fascinated. I had to do this. I had to be a homeopath. It seemed like magic, and yet it also seemed to make complete sense. There was a logic to it that seemed perfect. Homeopathy seemed to be able to heal people in a way that orthodox medicine could not even begin to emulate. (Further on I give a couple of examples from my early practice that did seem like magic.) Here I was, having spent two or three years reading about esoteric subjects from eastern Europe and India, sitting in the middle of London listening to lectures of the most extraordinary kind. And the lectures were being given by pillars of the establishment. Dr Marjorie Blackie was a physician to the Queen. I had heard doctors joke about homeopathic doses of drugs – usually when a medical student had suggested a dose that was far too small for a patient. The doses used in homeopathic medicine are incredibly small. No one was able to explain to me how homeopathy worked, but that didn't negate it in anyway as far as I was concerned. I felt quite sure that quantum physics would one day provide the explanation. In the nuclear age we can no longer be surprised at the properties of sub-atomic particles and energy waves.

What I found particularly fascinating was that the homeo-pathic medicine must exactly match the patient in order to have a healing effect. (I have always thought it something like the effect that a vibrating tuning fork has on another of similar frequency at the other end of a room.) This requires from the homeopath great sensitivity and receptivity to the patient, and a willingness not to expect answers immediately: a contrast to my formal medical education. I never looked back. I attended all the RLHH courses. I was particularly inspired by Dr Marjorie Blackie who was Dean at the Homoeopathic Hospital. As I was still a medical student at the time I started my homeopathic studies, I had to write to Dr Blackie and ask her permission to attend the lectures at the hospital. I was astonished when she telephoned me the next day and said 'Do come.'

I also started going to evening classes in homeopathy run by Thomas Maugham, who lived not very far from me. He was an extraordinary man, probably in his late sixties, who reminded me of Gurdjieff. His teaching was rather different from what I was learning at the Faculty of Homeopathy. His emphasis was on using homeopathy as a tool for assisting the evolution of the patient as a human being: 'evolutionary homeopathy' as it is sometimes called. I lost touch with

Thomas Maugham when I qualified as a doctor and moved down to Cornwall for my first hospital job. Some of his students went on to start the College of Homeopathy, the first training course for professional homeopaths in England.

Working in hospitals

Meanwhile I completed my medical degree, and then some junior hospital posts. I rarely mentioned homeopathy to the other doctors I was working with. Most doctors considered it a ridiculous thing to be doing, if not downright quackery. I really enjoyed working in hospitals. I enjoyed the buzz, the sense of achievement I got from getting through a lot of work efficiently and effectively. I enjoyed working with other people, the nursing staff, the other doctors and the patients. I enjoyed making the patients laugh. I also enjoyed the social life that revolved around living in the hospital, which was essential in those first two years. My first hospital post was in Cornwall. It was one of those long hot summers in the mid-1970s. Most of my evenings off I went to the beach with friends from work, or for a walk along the cliffs. It was a magical time. As I was working in acute surgery, many of the patients I saw were getting rapid relief from the surgical treatments they received: appendicectomies, the lancing of abscesses, removal of various lumps and bumps.

After this job, I moved back to London for posts in general medicine and then obstetrics. These posts I enjoyed too, although the nights on call began to pall after a while. I considered becoming a general physician, but then three years after qualifying as a doctor I sat the membership examinations for the Faculty of Homeopathy, which I passed. At about the same time I sat the Part 1 examination for membership of the Royal College of Physicians – all multiple choice questions. I had prepared well and thought that I knew enough of the answers to get a fairly good pass. But as I walked away from the examination hall I suddenly had a sinking feeling in my stomach. I realised that I had filled in the multiple choice computer slip incorrectly. I had gone straight down the column instead of across. This meant that except for question one all my answers would be in the wrong boxes. When the results came I found that I had failed so badly that I was not allowed to re-sit for three years. I had never failed an exam before. I took it as a sign, and shortly after, in September 1978, I set up my own private practice in homeopathy. I was soon inundated with patients.

Independent practice

Stepping out of the orthodox medical world – the NHS – was a big relief to me. There were many reasons for this. One was the very long working hours, and in particular frequent calls in the middle of the night. Often I would hardly get to bed all night and then would still have to work a full day. But most of all, I could now get on and practise medicine the way that I wanted. I wouldn't feel the need to hide my thoughts any longer. It might have been scary, but I didn't find it so. I had seen others being successful in private homeopathic practice, and felt quite confident that I would be also. I had really enjoyed working in hospitals, but it was time to move on, and practise in the way that I thought would be the most effective. It was not just about homeopathy. It was also about having time to listen to people, and to try and really understand the nature and causes of their 'dis-ease'.

My clinics were always full. People came to wait just in case someone didn't show up for their appointment. It was quite extraordinary. Dorothy Sheppard called her first book *The Magic of the Minimum Dose* (1938). It really did work like that. People were being healed in body, mind and spirit. Some of the results were truly remarkable. I remember one of my early cases, a young Jamaican woman with quite bad arthritis in both wrists. I gave her two doses of a homeopathic medicine called Pulsatilla, which is made from a plant of that name. I chose it because it was a good match for her in many different ways. When she came to see me again a month later, she said 'What was in those two pills you gave me? That night I had a bath and after I had finished bathing I just got out of the bath without thinking. I was really scared. Lord, I said, this is a miracle.' Normally she couldn't get out of the bath without assistance. Her pain had gone.

Another case concerned a woman with painful osteo-arthritis of 20 years duration. I gave her two doses of homeo-pathic Sulphur, which perfectly matched her symptoms and her constitution. When the woman came back a month or so later, she reported that she had been able to wash her hair herself for the first time in many years: 'I danced around the room saying "I've washed my hair, I've washed my hair!"' One of the wonderful things about homeopathy is that the treatment is not necessarily ongoing, even in chronic illness. Often a single dose of a similar homeopathic medicine (that is one that matches the patient in many different ways, and resonates with the person) is enough. But of course not everyone responded well. That is the great challenge of homeopathy: to find the cure for every case.

Teaching and further study

In 1979 I was asked to join the teaching team of the newly formed College of Homeopathy. I was to give the medical science lectures. I discovered that I enjoyed teaching immen-sely and after a few months I began teaching homeopathy also. Among the teachers and students at the college were people who were to become my closest friends. It was this group who were the founders of the Society of Homeopaths. It was a very exciting time. Everyone was thirsty for knowledge. Myself and others were looking for a teacher who could take us the next step. This man was to be George Vithoulkas.

Vithoulkas was a Greek engineer who came across homeopathy while working in South Africa. He came back to Greece and started the Centre for Homeopathic Medicine in Athens. In 1982 I saw a mention of his name in a health magazine which gave information about a seminar he was running on the Greek island of Alonissos. I noted down all the details and booked right away. It took two days to get there from London in those days. The seminar was held in the village school. There were about 30 delegates in all; most were American doctors. One American, Roger Morrison, had learned Greek specifically to spend a year sitting in with George. There was no one else from England. We were accommodated in rooms around the beautiful bay of Rossoum. The teaching was inspiring. It was the beginning of a new phase of learning for me.

At that time Vithoulkas taught only doctors, believing that only doctors were allowed to practise homeopathy (this was certainly the case in Greece). The following year I returned to Alonissos. This time there were doctors from all over Europe, but again no one from England except one who had been told he couldn't come because he wasn't a doctor. He came anyway. His persistence paid off. I later learned that Vithoulkas was not approved of in England because he wasn't a doctor. I told George that anyone could practise homeopathy in England, and the next year he gave a seminar for a large English group from the Society of Homeopaths.

Under pressure to come and teach in England, and reluctant to travel himself, Vithoulkas sent one of the teachers from his Athens clinic to give a series of lectures in England. This man was Vassilis Ghegas, a passionate and effusive Greek doctor, and a very knowledgeable homeopath. He gave freely of everything he knew. Vassilis would stay in London with an old friend of his from Ireland who he had met on a retreat many years before. His lectures were immensely popular.

During these weekends many of my homeopathic friends would come and stay in my London flat. We learned a lot, talked a lot, and drank plenty of wine. Being part of a world-wide community of passionate and dedicated homeopaths was exciting and challenging. There was so much to learn. Most of those that I mixed with were not doctors, but some were. I found that many of the doctors in the homeopathic world had difficulty in fully embracing the homeopathic model. They seemed too stuck in the model of orthodox medicine to be able to fully grasp the homeopathic way of thinking. This may have been simply to do with the way their minds worked after years of scientific training, or perhaps it was the time pressures of working within busy NHS practices. There were doctors who seemed able to do so, however. Some of these were later to become my partners in the Homeopathic Physicians Teaching Group (HPTG).

The excitement of being able to heal people in such a remarkable way continued to be tempered by the failures. The more I learned, the more difficult it seemed to improve my results further. Being a homeopath is certainly humbling. A year or so after Vassilis first came over, a small group of us formed the Academy of Classical Homeopathy, specifically to bring Vithoulkas over to England to teach. The aim was to work with live patients, all of whom had previously had homeopathic treatment that had been unsuccessful. We used a high quality video link to record the consultations, and to make them more private for the patient. I believe this was the first time that video recording was used in homeopathic education. Personality clashes and other difficulties led to the

programme being discontinued, but the model was established. Vithoulkas went on to found and build the International
Academy of Classical Homeopathy back on Alonissos where
he has his home.

Beyond homeopathy

I also became increasingly interested in other aspects of health:
healthy environment, lifestyle, food, and also other forms of
alternative medicine. I studied massage, soft tissue manipulation, orthobionomy, iridology, neurolinguistic programming,
and Erikssonian hypnosis. I learned yoga and aikido. I became
vegetarian, ate mostly wholefoods, and made fresh vegetable
and fruit juices using a Boots wine press. I went to seminars
about alternative methods of treating cancer, including the
Gerson method (a strict diet and juice therapy developed by Dr
Max Gerson, available at the Gerson Institute in San Diego,
California), and Laetrile (also known as Amygdalin, or vitamin
B17: it is extracted from apricot kernals. Laetrile is used as a
cancer treatment, and is championed by Dr Ernesto Contreras
at his clinic in Tijuana, Mexico). And of course I enjoyed life.
My passion for music which started at an early age has always
remained with me. I learned to play the flute and the violin. I
went to evening classes in traditional Irish music run by that
wild Irish fiddler and impresario Brendan Mulkere, and then
later to the Willy Clancy summer school of music at Milton
Malbay in the west of Ireland where I had tin whistle lessons
from Mary Bergin. If you like the tin whistle, Mary Bergin has
to be heard. Most of the traditional musicians in Ireland
seemed to be there for the week, teaching the classes and
playing in the pubs in the evenings. There seemed to be more
pubs than houses in the small town, but they were all packed.
    In the mid-1980s one of my friends made contact with an
Israeli homeopath called Joseph Reves and some of us started

going to his classes in England. He was a strict Hahnemanian homeopath whose teaching was mostly philosophy. We discussed homeopathic philosophy, explored new ideas and concepts of health and sickness. We explored the language that our patients use – how the simple language of the patient reveals their inner state and may guide you to the homeopathic medicine they need. We discussed the relationship between sensation and function and the law of the pipe (that what goes in must come out). All were different ways of trying access the inner being of the patient, not just his or her mind, but how the whole organism functioned, or failed to function in the world. It has been a never-ending source of wonder to me how the central disturbance in the vital force shows itself in symptoms of both mind and body, each symptom manifesting the disturbance in a different way, but still retaining the signature of the centre.

Around this time I sold my flat in London and moved to Malvern. Some friends had already started a small homeo-pathic philosophy study group there. After a year this group expanded considerably. A remarkable group of people had left the homeopathy college at which they were studying as they were dissatisfied with the standard of teaching. They set up a co-operative college known as the Darlington Collective and employed their own lecturers. Having completed their training, the Darlington Collective joined together with the Malvern Group for ongoing postgraduate study. It was from this group that the Dynamis School arose.

The Dynamis School has become a magnet for those wanting to take their studies of homeopathy to another dimen-sion. The two-year course is philosophy based, and central to the learning there is participating in provings (the testing of homeopathic medicines to determine their properties). There is nothing like participating in provings for deepening your understanding of the hidden powers of medicines, the homeopathic process, and the interconnection of all things in the universe. It is in a sense the inner game of homeopathy. The most remarkable things happen during provings, but they require close observation or you may miss them altogether.

I shall always be grateful to Jeremy for showing me the way to the next level. It was through Jeremy and the Malvern Group that I met Dee. She was a founder member of the Darlington Collective and a brilliant homeopath. We had a good connection from our first meeting, but it was at a Dynamis retreat on the Hebridean island of Raasay that it seemed that we would become lovers. I was extremely resistant. I had not had a long-term relationship previously, and I was very clear that if I stepped into this one there would be no going back. The fireball dinghy that I had towed all the way from Devon to Rasaay tipped Dee into the water within seconds of leaving the shore. The dinghy's name was Aphrodite; I think she was jealous. I nearly blew it. It was only after telling Dee that it wouldn't work that I realised I didn't want to live without her. We have been together ever since; it was the best decision I have ever made.

A time of illness

It was after windsurfing on a reservoir that I developed a fever. I felt colder inside than I had ever felt before in my life, and I ached all over. I also had extreme lassitude, everything seemed too much effort. It lasted for a few days, and then I seemed to have recovered, but the symptoms kept on coming back. One week I would be perfectly alright, and then the next week I felt as if I had a bad dose of flu. This went on for months, and then years. I learned to live with it, and I was able to carry on working part time. Homeopathic treatment wasn't helping. I began reading widely searching for a cure. I read about food sensitivities, gut dysbiosis and leaky gut syndrome. I started to read extensively about supplements: vitamins, minerals, anti-oxidants, essential fatty acids, enzymes, etc. I had all the various tests done on myself. There was nothing conclusive, but over the years I was gradually improving.

Finally I met a man called Adrian Lindeman who specialises in the diagnosis of hidden infections using a vega machine, which measures electrical resistance at accupuncture points on the skin. He treats the infections he finds using nosodes – homeopathic doses of the infecting organisms. Among other things he diagnosed me as having an amoebic liver abscess (I had suffered amoebic dysentery in India in 1976). Within a few days of starting the treatment people were telling me that I no longer looked yellow, and I was gradually restored to full health. Lindeman's method is at the opposite end of the spectrum from classical homeopathy. He certainly opened my eyes to another way of working with potentised medicines. I have found it to be very effective in precisely cases like my own (known nowadays as post-viral chronic fatigue syndrome). Lindeman is a most unusual man. Previously an engineer in South Africa, he has dedicated his life to his work with nosodes. He designs and builds machines for detecting illness, makes his own nosode medicines, and does much research on unusual viruses and other pathogenic organisms.

I continued to search for more information about how to treat and prevent chronic disease. In recent years much of my searching has been done on the internet, which has given me more rapid access to the kind of information that I have been seeking. So much chronic illness is simply accelerated ageing, the result of poor nutrition and a sedentary lifestyle. This has led me into the field of anti-ageing medicine and life extension. I discovered that an enormous amount of research is being done throughout the world in this field. Much of this research has been collated, mostly in the United States, and protocols have been developed for slowing down and even reversing many of the ageing processes. By synergistic application of several strategies, remarkable results can be achieved. I used many of the various disciplines I had studied in my practice, but I had to learn more.

My work with anti-ageing medicine is now an integral part of my everyday practice. It really is possible to slow down the degenerative effects of ageing. Infirmity and diminished cognitive function are no longer a necessary part of getting old. I have also set up a company called Anti-Ageing Technologies for people who don't necessarily have a specific health problem, but who wish to discover how to slow down ageing. Consultations include a full medical and lifestyle assessment, together with wide-ranging investigations to determine real age as compared to chronological age. By having clear markers of how much ageing damage has already been done, it is much easier to assess how much real progress is being made, other than just feeling better. Many people of course opt for feeling better without necessarily wanting to have all the tests.

The Homeopathic Physicians Teaching Group

Shortly after Jeremy Sherr had started the Dyanamis School, I got together with others to start a homeopathy college for doctors. We were a group of like-minded homeopathic doctors who were dissatisfied with the education in homeopathy that was currently available in England. Many of us had studied with George Vithoulkas on Alonissos, but not all at the same time. Eight of us founded the HPTG (then known as the Homeopathic Physicians Teaching Group) in 1993. The three-year part-time training course that we set up was to provide more than double the contact teaching hours of any other course for doctors, had a carefully structured curriculum, guided home study, and regular regional tutorial groups. We attracted students from all over the country, and also some from abroad, including Ireland and the United States. One of the most successful features of our course was the residential modules. By staying overnight students would have time to socialise with their peers, and many have developed long-lasting friendships and support group networks as a result. The regional tutorial groups served a similar purpose.

All of the HPTG teaching partners meet regularly in a group with a psychotherapist to air their feelings, mostly about what is happening in the HPTG, but not exclusively so. This I believe to be one of the reasons the partnership has held together so well. One of our number died in a tragic accident, two others have left, but we have retained a strong core. Four years after the founding of the HPTG, the UK veterinary homeopathic course joined us and became amalgamated into our main course. The union has introduced a fascinating new dimension into the teaching of homeopathy. The doctors have learned much from the vets, and vice versa. Of the three veterinary tutors that joined us, two eventually became partners, and have become part of the essential core of the HPTG. Two further developments include postgraduate supervision groups with regular training in supervision for the tutors, and also a teacher training programme, which nine HPTG graduates participated in. Five of these have been regular lecturers on the course over the past year. The HPTG has also extended overseas, and is currently running a veterinary course in Australia and in Ireland. Future possibilities include courses in the United States and Japan.

The future

The future looks very exciting from my perspective. Our knowledge of how to slow ageing, and to heal the sick in both mind and body is advancing fast. Some of these advances are simply in our knowledge of what constitutes good nutrition for a human being. Our bodies can get away with a lot, but at the end of the day, eating poor quality food will have an effect. Modern food is adulterated in so many different ways. It is damaged by heat (cooking), grown in mineral deficient soil and sprayed with chemicals or, in the case of animals, fed an unnatural diet and pumped full of hormones. By choosing carefully what we eat we can make a huge difference to the quality of our lives.

At the other end of the spectrum we have made numerous very high tech advances. We now have the possibility of curing diseases caused by genetic malformations. Stem cell research is very far advanced. Reversing Parkinson's Disease by stem cell implantation may not be far away. A similar cure for insulin dependent diabetes is just around the corner. In a few years we will be able to grow new teeth to replace rotten ones. Don't have that implant, just wait a bit. So what do I enjoy most about my work? I love the thrill of new discoveries, new possibilities to improve people's quality of life, and being an information resource to direct my patients to the latest methods. For some reason it can take years for advances in medicine to filter through to GPs. I love exchanging my knowledge with others: with my peers and with my students. I love the interaction with my patients, the detective work involved in searching for the root causes of their problems, and the dance of matching my recommendations for them with their perception of what they want and how they want to proceed. I love to see the dawning realisation in my patients that they have a new life ahead of them. Now that's magic.

Conclusion

After nearly 30 years in medicine I have come to the conclusion that no one system has all the answers. Both orthodox medicine and most systems of complementary medicine have something to offer, some perhaps more than others. It is not an easy task to separate what is likely to be helpful from what might be harmful, either in itself or by omission, in any particular case. What is crucial is to really listen to the patient, to try to understand their wishes, needs, fears and anxieties, and to explore with them the various therapeutic options that might be available to them.

Every patient is unique and each one brings a new and fresh challenge to the doctor. Being mindful of this in every case is an opportunity for the doctor to bring his or her passion for life into the consulting room and perhaps help the patient rediscover their own.

References

Sheppard, D. (1938) *The Magic of the Minimum Dose.* London: Homoeopathic Publishing Co.

Introduction to Chapter 7

The main theme running through Charles Forsyth's piece is epitomised in his two quotes at the beginning. He seems to have been searching for answers ever since adolescence. Medical training was not as traumatic for him as for many of the other authors, but like them he often felt lonely and unsupported and wonders if more support could not be given to newly qualified doctors.

When I asked Charles what was the most important message he would like the reader to take away from his writing, his reply was:

> Life is a journey and every moment of that journey is an unrivalled opportunity for us to learn (and love) more about ourselves, others and the universe we find ourselves in – for us to wake up.

I was reminded of the quote at the beginning of Alice Greene's chapter which also begins with an exhortation to wake up. It seems to be the message of all the great spiritual teachers and seems a fitting end to the book.

Chapter 7

My Journey into Medicine
Charles Forsyth

Two Shakespearean quotes have been major threads running
through my life:

> This above all, to thine own self be true,
> And it must follow as the night the day
> Thou canst not then be false to any man.

Hamlet: Act 1, Scene III

> There are more things in heaven and earth, Horatio,
> Than are dreamt of in your philosophy.

Hamlet: Act 1, Scene V

My journey into medicine has been inextricably intertwined
with my own personal journey, which seems to be about my
struggle from darkness and half-truths into light, the shedding
of veils, a voyage of discovery: that of myself and my place in
the universe.

Early life

My parents thought I would be an engineer. I loved to know how things worked and was good with my hands. At school it was the sciences that caught my imagination and the sheer beauty of nature and its laws filled me with wonder and excitement. At the same time I had an emotionally challenging childhood. My parents were northerners who moved south to Portsmouth when my father took a short commission in the Navy. They were both dentists, having trained at Leeds dental school. My mother didn't find babies and young children easy and openly admitted that she only really liked children when they could read and hold discussions. Later, seeing her with my babies was hugely revealing; she just didn't know how to relate to them on an instinctive level. No wonder I had difficulty with close emotional relationships. She was a complex soul: on the one hand a passionate and enthusiastic woman who enjoyed socialising and on the other an intellectual. She loved argument, literature and the arts and had strong views about many areas, especially education and women's causes. However, she lacked a basic confidence in herself and was hopeless at showing affection. My father, on the other hand, was sporty, loved cricket and rugby and taught me to play squash. I had a much closer relationship with him although it must have been frustrating for him that I was not sportier. I think my mother was allergic to exercise and couldn't understand my father's rather 'fidgety' nature. It is interesting that my love of exercise and activity only emerged quite a lot later in my life.

My mother returned to work soon after my birth and I was looked after by a series of nannies. The last one, Ivy, a spinster, gave me some of the mother-love that I had desperately lacked. At eight I was sent away to boarding school and life changed abruptly. I suspect I still don't know the full impact this had on me, but I adapted, I got on with life. My school reports referred to me as being idle and lazy but this seemed to disappear around the age of ten. I think that it was at that time that I learnt to 'perform' – to meet other people's expectations at the cost of being more out of touch with my inner world. For years I dreaded the beginning of term. Several days before, the trunk would come out for packing and this signalled the journey back to the other life. But once I was dropped off, the last one was soon forgotten. My ability to forget the past too quickly, not reflect on it, or learn from it and integrate it, took another turn for the worse.

At 12 I was sent to a 'crammer' for two terms to get me through Common Entrance. What a change this was: from a school of 100 boys to one of 30, all the same age and there because we were either thick, lazy or naughty! It was a very different atmosphere; we were given much more respect and responsibility and there was a clear relationship between pulling one's weight with the work, and the privilege of being there. There was a very firm strictness but a caring attitude. This was growing up.

The transition to public school was another big leap. It was in my early days there, the first term probably, that I learnt to laugh and smile in the face of fear/threats/danger. I remember one particular event clearly. I was being set upon by a number of boys and I discovered that with laughter I could give the impression I was stronger and braver than I really was, so I was left alone, relatively unchallenged. This is my first recollection of a feeling of aloofness. This may have started earlier at prep school, but it was another large notch marking a yet further separation of the outer life I lived, my fragile façade, from my true inner feelings, a pattern that was to continue for most of my life.

When I was about 15 I became aware that my parents' relationship was in difficulty and they discussed with my brother and me the possibility of them separating. I can't remember my response, or whether the possibility had occurred to me before this. Being away at school, I had been sheltered from virtually all of what had been going on. I had always been aware of the arguments and 'bad vibes', but it was only much later on that I realised how much I had blocked off this atmosphere of unspoken anger, frustration and resentment, yet how much it coloured my life. A few days before my sixteenth birthday, my father committed suicide.

Once back at school, it was really as if nothing had happened. My house master was understanding but my recollection is that the matter was hardly mentioned, and I received only one letter from a friend of the family offering me emotional support, which I didn't take up. I look back in amazement – I shed virtually no tears, I experienced almost no grief – over the one person in my life who I felt closest to and had a genuine emotional connection with. I just got on with it, one door closing, another opening, and no reflection. My father had just cut himself off, as surely as anyone can, from his feelings and here I was doing the same. How very much we learn to do this as doctors, so that we can 'do our job' and not be too affected. 'Put on your armour' is a phrase that I remember from medical school.

Dawning of consciousness

Around this time my life at Malvern College took an abrupt turn. I found two books on Buddhism in the school library. I can clearly remember one of them having an orange cover and being full of Buddhist aphorisms. I also started practising some yoga. They must have had quite a profound effect, for suddenly another dimension had opened up for me. There was a level of consciousness beyond normal everyday consciousness. It was as if I was emerging from a sleep. I was more awake, more aware, the scales were dropping from my eyes and I was seeing, hearing, sensing with a new clarity – as if everything was more in focus, was more real, more fresh, more alive. This was living!

I had the great good fortune to be at a school that was in the Malvern Hills where I could escape into the most beautiful natural surroundings. My love of nature, art and music escalated. There was a great sense of freedom and potential. I developed a distrust of conventional Western wisdom and wanted little to do with conservative society. However, I managed to toe the line with my education. I was taking biology, chemistry and physics at 'A' Level and thoroughly enjoying them. In fact, my appreciation of the natural world exploded and I was filled with wonder, delight, amazement and awe at nature from the microscopic to the cosmic. My reading broadened and I discovered the following lines by William Wordsworth around this time.

> And I have felt
> A presence that disturbs me with the joy
> Of elevated thoughts: a sense sublime
> Of something far more deeply interfused,
> Whose dwelling is the light of setting suns,
> And the round ocean and the living air,
> And the blue sky, and in the mind of man;
> A motion and a spirit, that impels
> All thinking things, all objects of all thought,
> And rolls through all things.
>
> *Tintern Abbey, 1798*

The darkness was becoming much less dark, shafts of light shone in, and at last I had a sense of direction and purpose: something had really touched my innermost being.

The decision to go into medicine just seemed to happen. I can't remember agonising too much about what I wanted to do, or even any lengthy discussions. I think I was fairly disinterested, and I certainly had no idea what I wanted to do, either in the short or long term, regarding an occupation. I was finally enjoying life and would have been more than happy to have continued with my wanderings, picking up odd jobs here and there, and living a nice hippy existence. I loved the sciences, so it seemed appropriate to do something along those lines, but what? The idea of laboratory work did not appeal. I had a good vocational guidance assessment, which suggested that something to do with people would be appropriate. Then medicine was mentioned as a possibility: it fulfilled all the criteria, it kept my options open and I could move into purer sciences later if I wanted to. And that was it. I didn't have the confidence, self-assuredness or clarity to follow my own path. Maybe just as well!

Beginning medical school and exploring spirituality

My feelings about my first year at medical school were mixed. I didn't want to be tied down. I found no students on my wavelength and felt like a fish out of water. I had chosen to go into digs as I saw the hall of residence as no different from the institutionalised living which I had just escaped. The trouble was that I had been given a family to live with who I regarded as boringly conventional in what might have been considered as the pits of London: Catford, way away from the centre. So began an extremely lonely, but formative year. What it gave me was plenty of time for reflection on myself. I had been thrust into my own inner world for the first time, to confront my feelings, which were dominated by sadness and depression. I practised yoga regularly and instinctively knew meditation was what I was looking for. But what type of meditation and what path was right for me?

This was the year that I consciously started spiritually searching, looking at Buddhism, especially Zen and Tibetan, Sufism, Subud, etc. I discovered Hermann Hesse and was deeply moved by his book *Siddhartha* (1998). Meanwhile at medical school I enjoyed the basic medical sciences but found most of the teaching very dry and lacking enthusiasm for the wonders of science and the human body. The end of my first year saw me on the road (yet) again. One of my destinations was Findhorn, a new age spiritual community started in the sixties by Peter and Eileen Caddy, near Inverness in Scotland. This was a visit that was to change my life, forever. For the first time I was with people who actually shared my spiritually questing nature. My visit had been spontaneous and, as it happened, there was an international conference on 'Consciousness and Education', which had drawn people from all over the world. This proved to be a real highlight in my life; I felt an incredible depth of openness, love, clarity and purity. I took a great liking to a couple that I met there, who extolled the virtues of homeopathy and were following a spiritual path with an Indian teacher. I had become initiated into transcendental meditation as it was something practical and accessible that I could get on with, but it didn't really hit the spot. What surprises me looking back is the lack of depth of my spiritual research. It was as if at some level I knew what I was looking for and I would know it when I found it. It was as if the aroma was enough to tell whether it was right or not.

Then one day I was reading the book *Path of the Masters* one of the books about the path that my friends were following and it was as if a light had suddenly come on. A window or door to a whole new world just opened up, and the pieces of a huge jigsaw puzzle suddenly fell into place. Tears flowed, seemingly endlessly. I knew that I had found what I had been looking for. This, at last, was a philosophy that made perfect sense: on the one hand to my intellect, and on the other, to my intuition. It put forward a unified hypothesis that explained the physical, emotional, mental and spiritual worlds, the nature of man, life and death: all the paranormal phenomena that I was interested in, the path to enlightenment and the puzzling diversity of religions seeking the same spiritual truths. At the same time it felt absolutely right; it had a deep resonance within me. What was more, it stated that there was always at least one real living teacher on the planet who had attained the highest levels of consciousness, and that there was one at present living in the Punjab in India.

Beginning work with patients

In 1974 I started my clinical training and medicine really began for me. Patients, the wards, ward rounds, learning about diseases, blood taking, sitting in on clinics, surgical theatres, A&E, consultants and their teams, the nursing staff, etc. Exciting times, so much to learn, so much to do. Everything became practical, everything patient focused. This was new – no longer just the joy of understanding for understanding's sake, it was now intensely humanised: to do with relationships. What a refreshing change. I had great fondness, respect and admiration for my consultants while at the same time being quietly amused by their old-school manner. Interestingly, I did not find the experience at all traumatic or in any conflict with my nature. I took to it without difficulty and did not have expectations of it being any different from how it was. Somehow my alternative, spiritual viewpoint was not challenged, not that I felt the need to talk about it, and I felt part of a caring team. There was a great feeling of warmth and of everyone pulling together.

The next year my medical elective was due, and the question was, where to spend it? India, of course! Somewhere close to my spiritual path. I was fortunate to be accepted by the Postgraduate Institute of Medical Education and Research (PGI), Chandigarh, for a two-month attachment, and also by the spiritual centre for a visit.

Another life-changing moment. As I stepped out of the plane at Delhi airport, I was suddenly overwhelmed with tears and a feeling of being completely and utterly, back home. Such a sense of familiarity, love and comfort that I had never experienced anywhere else before just rushed into me. My two months at PGI were not particularly helpful medically as I was the only undergraduate in a centre where all the postgraduates were eager for experience, I was left pretty much to myself, did not push myself forward and really just hung around. However, two weeks spent at a small rural hospital was an experience of real India. My visit to the Dera, just outside the village of Beas, on the banks of the Beas river (one of the five main rivers of the Punjab) was out of this world. The master, Charan Singh, defied description. He had all and more of the qualities that I had read about belonging to a true master. Visiting India, being with followers of this path and actually having ten days in the presence of a living master, was truly a coming home.

Finding medical freedom

A year later I met my future wife, Georgina, who was a third-year student nurse at Guy's Hospital with me, and the following year I succeeded in qualifying. I enjoyed my house jobs but found the first one in general medicine very stressful as I received very little support. In retrospect, I think it would be a good idea to build more support in the form of mentoring into the profession, particularly as a part of the first year. I know teachers have begun to take on this form of support to reduce rates of burnout and I think it would be a good idea for doctors to do the same. But I must point out that this may of course be the case now: it was in 1977 that I started my first house job.

It was a steep learning curve, but I was doctoring! Next I did an A&E job which satisfied my practical nature and I was gaining experience and some independence. After a few locums, Georgina and I married and we went to New Zealand for a year's working holiday/honeymoon. Locum work as a GP was plentiful and I just loved it. Then another awakening took place. My new-found medical independence gave me a completely new perspective. Now that it was entirely my responsibility how I managed my patients and what I prescribed for them, I started to think more deeply about them and how I cared for them. Why are they getting sick: what are the real reasons for their pathologies? Is the treatment that I'm offering really addressing causes? What role could their diet and nutrition be playing? I had a strong suspicion that stress and one's psychological make-up played a vital role in so much ill health. I was drawn to look at my patients with a greater depth and breadth to make real sense of their disease process. But I had not been trained to do this type of holistic assessment and diagnosis. I also felt that the therapeutic tools I had been trained to use were very inadequate for what I wanted to achieve and clearly couldn't address more fundamental causes. They were sufficient to bail people out of crises and to some extent to containing chronic diseases, but I sensed that if I really wanted to make a positive difference to people's health and happiness, particularly in the long term, I had to look elsewhere.

I was seriously attracted to psychotherapy but at the same time I recognised that in my role as a doctor it was not going to be much use in most emergency situations. I had to have some therapy that was powerful enough to cope rapidly, effectively and safely with medical emergencies and deep enough to address real causes. I felt that nutrition was very important, but knew very little about it as I had received no significant training in the subject at medical school. However, I felt it did not really get right to the root of disease. Homeopathy raised its head again. Previously I had not given training in it another thought. How on earth would I want to submit to a another long and arduous training so soon after completing five years at medical school and a year of house jobs? But I knew that I could not continue to practise medicine in a way that was not holistic, did not deal with the causes as well as their effects, did not openly examine a patient's whole state and which had such a restricted range of interventions.

Instinctively I was drawn to homeopathy. From the little I knew about it, it just felt right. Strangely, I was not attracted to acupuncture, nor for that matter, manipulative therapies, even though they would all have matched my practical and technical nature. For a while, as a house surgeon I had considered specialising in surgery, but couldn't bear the idea of being trapped in an operating theatre most of my life. I suspect that I also knew that it would not satisfy this deeper aspect of me.

Georgina and I returned prematurely from our overland trip home, due to my wife suffering a recurrence of hepatitis in Singapore. Within a week of our return to the UK I found myself at the Faculty on a two-day introductory course in homeopathy. What a complete revelation it was for me to be in a room together with 30 or 40 other doctors, all having questions and ideas along similar lines to mine. What a joy! Whilst we were away in New Zealand my mother-in-law had developed severe rheumatoid arthritis and I began a search for someone to treat her. I was recommended to Dr Farley Spink and arranged to visit and sit in on a session with him at his practice in Surrey. To my complete and utter surprise he made me an offer to join him as an apprentice! I was not even job hunting and at that stage had no idea what I was going to do next.

We had two months before I was due to start a paediatric job that I had accepted before we left the UK and I was not at all sure that this was what I now wanted. I had had lots of experience in a wide variety of GP settings, both rural and urban, in New Zealand and felt that going back to hospital work would be unbearable – like having my wings clipped. I was very tempted to emigrate to New Zealand: we had had such a wonderful time and it would fulfil my love of outdoor life and my sense of freedom. However, learning another system of medicine would have been impossible, as there were hardly any homeopaths, let alone a training course in the country. Working in Croydon and settling in Surrey was certainly not what I had in mind either, but if I was to train in homeopathy, this seemed an ideal opportunity. After much deliberation I decided to go for it.

A new beginning

So started a difficult few years. I had not realised how different life would be. I was suddenly a fish out of water again. Almost all my old medical friends dropped away from me as if I were a leper. I wasn't in the familiar GP setting with the respect and friendship of local colleagues and I was therapeutically impotent! I was thrown in at the deep end, seeing patients from day one. They came seeking skills I did not yet possess and had no interest in the ones I did have. I was totally dependent on my trainer to prescribe on the notes that I had taken without him even seeing the patients. I sat in on his sessions, received teaching from him, attended the courses at the Royal London Homeopathic Hospital and did as much reading as I could muster. I have to admit, I found the latter extremely dry and unexciting, especially as reading has never been my preferred method of learning. I felt alone again. In 1981 there were not that many homeopathic doctors and we were very widely dispersed. The Faculty of Homeopathy was not as community minded and supportive as it is now. Georgina and I were finding our feet again after a year of travel and she was only slowly recovering from hepatitis. I too was probably not 100 per cent healthy, as I also had hepatitis and when I am stressed and my confidence is knocked, I tend to go into my shell. However, in May 1982 I sat and passed the examinations for membership of the Faculty of Homeopathy (MFHom). I was now a homeopath, at least a novice one!

Then the next revelation happened: George Vithoulkas and Vassilis Ghegas started teaching in London, thanks to the Society of Homeopaths. This was an inspiration to me – exciting, experienced, dynamic homeopaths with a new slant. Also meeting up with a wonderfully diverse and enthusiastic group of (non-medical) homeopaths: more like-minded souls. I had been struggling with homeopathy. At that point the remedies seemed to me to be just a collection of symptoms with no common thread that ran through them, no sense of cohesion and I had no real understanding of them. The 'remedy picture' had been evolving during the past 100 years but still lacked a depth that I felt should be there. Now Vithoulkas was offering us his concept of 'essence', that there is often a basic dynamic that is characteristic of, and runs through, the remedy picture, and is expressed in the symptoms. I instinctively felt this was getting closer to what I was seeking, albeit mostly subconsciously. This was exciting. I felt I was getting closer to the truth, something more central and fundamental. These seminars stretched over a couple of years or so and for me culminated in 1984, when I attended one of his seminars on the island of Alonissos in Greece, together with most of the homeopaths who had been attending the London seminars. It was at this course that George suggested we form a core group to train as teachers and then train other teachers. Unfortunately, this venture collapsed in its infancy due to personality clashes.

Alongside homeopathy, I started using nutritional approaches in my practice in the very early eighties. I had come into contact with and attended courses run by Dr Stephen Davies, one of the pioneers of nutritional medicine in the UK. There were few nutritional investigations, apart from conventional ones, available at the time, but this was soon to change, thanks to Stephen and Dr John McLaren Howard, who was a biochemist at the London Clinic and was the first in the country to offer hair element analysis. The pair teamed up in 1984 to found Biolab, a medical laboratory specialising in investigations relating to nutritional status. The same year I was a founder member of the British Society for Nutritional Medicine, which later amalgamated with the British Society for Allergy and Environmental Medicine, to become the British Society for Allergy, Environmental and Nutritional Medicine.

The year 1985 brought a wonderful new focus to my life, with the birth of our first child, Thomas. But it was a real struggle to find a balance between the demands of parenting and home life, my work, and my spiritual path. In 1987 I ventured further afield and did a course in electro-acupuncture. I had been fascinated by Chinese medicine, but had never taken it further; this was a chance to have an introduction without going too deep. As it turned out, I practised very little of what I had learnt, but it gave me a new understanding and perspective that I found helpful. A couple of years later the same was true of another venture, this time vega testing (a modified form of electro-acupuncture developed by the German doctor Voll in the 1950s). And in this same year my lovely daughter Jessica was born.

A big change in my clinical practice came later that year when I bought my first computer, an Apple Mac, to run one of the first serious homeopathic programs, MacRepertory. At last I was able to do homeopathic repertorisations (the process of using the homeopathic repertory to discover which homeopathic medicine covers the patient's symptoms best) almost instantly, something we all wanted to do, but found impossible in the usual busy clinic situation. However, my life was getting increasingly tough and I was plagued by fatigue, depression, migraines and irritable bowel syndrome. The following year I made the questionable decision to give up the struggle of trying to meditate for an hour or more daily. I went from one extreme to the other and stopped meditating altogether, rather than reduce it to a briefer period! This was part of a big swing away from being so intense and strict with myself, to taking life in a more relaxed fashion for the next few years. I was becoming quite disillusioned with homeopathy as a source of sorting out my own health problems, but I did benefit greatly from a variety of elimination diets, particularly sugar and yeast (the so called anti-candida diet), wheat/gluten and milk. But I did not have the self-discipline to stick to them and did not try desensitisation/neutralisation techniques (I suspected they were suppressive since they didn't deal with underlying causes). This was when my keen interest in gut function developed.

Professional friendship and support

In 1991 I was asked by colleagues if I would be interested in creating an undergraduate course in homeopathy. Now this was difficult to resist! I empathised greatly with prospective homeopathic students as I had found the task of getting to grips with the subject a real struggle. What a great group of doctors: almost all of us were of similar vintage and background, and keen to push the boundaries of medicine, homeopathy, healing and teaching further. Like-minded souls to work with! The following year we formed the Homeopathic Physicians Teaching Group (HPTG), based in Oxford and had our first intake of students. It was great fun, but very hard work and a steep learning curve. I had never taught before and most of us doubted our abilities and so over-prepared, as if we were teaching postgraduates.

We aimed to make our course everything we wished our own training had been: fun, dynamic, enthusiastic, clear, relevant, interactive, with plenty of group work and role-play and whole-person orientated. It was a delight to help doctors not only learn homeopathy but also undergo a paradigm shift in their view of medicine and life in general. The group also brought a real sense of belonging. This was the first group of professionals I had had such a close relationship with, people who shared similar core values and goals, and where there was mutual respect, support and understanding combined with a great sense of camaraderie.

I also saw the course as an opportunity to diversify, to cut back a bit on my clinical work and develop another source of income that was not dependent on patient consultations. At the same time, however, I was approached by Boots and offered the job of designing the homeopathic software for an in-store computer system to assist their customers in choosing appropriate homeopathic medicines. Another offer that I couldn't refuse at the time! The combination of both these projects brought me rapidly to my knees, working weekend after weekend on top of what was an already busy week in the clinic, and so started my mid-life crisis with a vengeance. I turned to psychotherapy rather than psychoanalysis and for the first time really started to face my inner demons.

Over the next couple of years my physical energy soared and I started doing all manner of outdoor activities, including cycling, running, kayaking, climbing and mountaineering, as well as returning to my old love of walking. This culminated in the most wonderful month-long trek with my best friend Peter in north east Nepal. Another joy was that I also found that dancing came naturally to me for the first time in my life, and music with rhythm became irresistible! I gradually began letting my hair down in a variety of ways, including drinking alcohol and smoking, having been a confirmed teetotaller and non-smoker for 15 years. The pent-up energy of the driven, restless, dissatisfied me was now finding an outlet physically, but I still had a ridiculous lack of confidence in myself.

I slowly came to realise a number of things about myself. I had not been recognising, let alone looking after my own needs. I was aware of others' needs far more than my own, and found that this in turn was really to attract care, love and attention to myself. How common this is amongst the caring professions! Sadly, it is really only the psychotherapists, as part of their training and professional life, who examine the dynamics underlying their therapeutic relationships. I passion-ately believe that we need to look at the reasons we do what we do, and how we do them. So many of us are in caring roles because of the care we didn't receive when we were very young. *Physician heal thyself.* And I certainly was in need of a lot of healing! I now recognised that when I didn't get the attention and love I craved, this was when I became depressed, forlorn, despondent or angry and resentful. I had been carry-ing a deep sense of sadness, emptiness and aloneness from very early childhood and had been avoiding these feelings by escaping into my head, developing my intellectual under-standing of the world, busying myself with outer activities and spiritually questing. I had almost completely shut off my feelings and to a large extent, my body.

Another pattern that I discovered was that I had a strong tendency to go to extremes; moderation or the middle way was a lovely idea, but didn't seem to be in my nature. A number of other big changes took place. I was no longer content to pretend I was feeling something when I wasn't. I was fed up with acting and portraying an image that was not true to the me inside. Whereas previously I had had huge difficulties dealing with my anger, now I was expressing it much more readily. Unfortunately, the pendulum swung too far the other way for quite a while and my poor wife took the brunt of it. My determination to survive and seek the truth served me well, but were not balanced by a place of inner calm, quietness and clarity. I gradually found myself wanting more time alone to be with my own thoughts and feelings and to find stillness within. I started to meditate again.

Meanwhile further exciting changes were taking place in homeopathy. Three leading lights appeared on the scene: Jan Scholten, Massimo Mangialavori and Rajan Sankaran. Jan, a homeopathic physician from Holland, has brought revolutionary homeopathic insight into the periodic table of the elements. For the first time, this offers the possibility of predicting aspects of an element's remedy picture just from its position in the table. He is also working on a similar model for the plant kingdom (see www.alonnissos.org). Massimo, a homeopathic physician from Italy, has devised the concept of 'themes', particularly within remedy families, such as sea creatures, snakes and insects. He has also brought a very high degree of rigour to the assessment of cured cases (see www.mangialavori.com/indeng.htm). Rajan, a homeopathic physician from India, has been developing and expanding the concept of miasms and remedy relationships within the three kingdoms of nature and is also developing a 'periodic table of plants' (see www.thespiritofhomoeopathy.com). These and other homeopaths have been contributing to a deep shift in homeopathy, a huge advance in its theory and practice, science and art.

Homeopathy is, on the one hand, coming closer to becoming a true science, with the ability to make more accurate predictions from more reliable models, and on the other hand is more consciously recognising, respecting and developing the role of intuition in what we do. I view this as an important aspect of true holism. As I see it, all truly great people have well developed, finely tuned minds and hearts. They are as sharp, critical and incisive with their intuition as they are in their thinking.

In the HPTG we felt strongly about the importance of group process and had a Freudian psychoanalyst facilitate sessions for the partners on a regular basis. This gave us a safe setting to explore and manage negative feelings that arose in the course of our work together. Later on we recognised the need for supervision; a concept alien to doctors and homeopaths at the time. We organised day-long group supervision sessions for ourselves also on a regular basis. Both of these group activities have helped us be a very cohesive supportive group, and have facilitated our growth, both as a group and as individuals. I warmed to teaching rapidly and enjoyed sharing my enthusiasm for the subjects that I loved. But it proved an interesting struggle to let go of my need to know everything, to be sure of my facts, my fears of being found out – and relax into sharing what I *did* know in a much more right-brained way.

Conclusion: connecting with patients and myself

One of the things that has changed so much for me in my practice in recent years is the level of connection I am able to develop with my patients. I have long felt that our ability to help our patients is both dependent on, and limited by, our own personal development, not only our degree of knowledge and experience. I believe we need to be fully and consciously engaged in our own personal growth process. I am sure this would benefit our patients. I also wonder about the personal and professional cost of not building in more time for reflection both in our training and practices. Real health is an ideal, a concept that we are moving towards. Making the subconscious conscious, being in tune with all levels of our being – physically, emotionally, mentally and spiritually – are part of this move. And ill health and disease can be our clearest guides on the path of personal growth. Our body/system is giving us messages constantly and most of the time we look the other way. The more we ignore our body, the more loudly it complains, until we take notice – or die.

We, as doctors/healers/therapists, are in the wonderfully enviable position of having the raw material of people to work with daily, exploring them (as well as ourselves) to whatever level we and they are prepared to go. Gradually, I am learning to be a more attentive practitioner, to be quieter, calmer and less busy inside so that I can be more receptive and open to the patient before me. And also open to myself: noticing when counter-transference/projective identification is taking place, and being able to make use of it in the session. I want all my faculties to be functioning as optimally as possible, and to do that I have to know myself, identify and resolve my own issues, be open to all possibilities and of course care for myself. My two favourite quotes from *Hamlet* are still guiding stars. It is a wonderful privilege to help others and relieve suffering, but to be involved in real healing and homeopathy demands more and more conscious engagement in the process of personal transformation, and this is magical.

References

Hesse, H. (1998) *Siddhartha*. New York: Picador. Translated by H. Rosner.

Johnson, J. (1985) *Path of the Masters*. India: Radha Soamisatsang Beas.

Contributors

David Curtin has been in full-time private practice as a homeopathic physician since 1978. He studied medicine at Guy's Hospital, and then homeopathy at the Royal London Homeopathic Hospital. Over the years he has studied widely to improve his understanding of homeopathy, key influences being George Vithoulkas, Jeremy Sherr and Rajan Sankaran. Since 1980 he has taught at several colleges of homeopathy in England and Ireland, has lectured internationally and was one of the founding members of the Oxford Group (HPTG). David has found that no one system of medicine has all the answers, and has developed an integrated approach which combines the best of orthodox and complementary medicine. Until recently he was Medical Director at the Integrated Medical Centre in London. Currently he is working in the NHS where he is undergoing further training in orthodox medicine.

Charles Forsyth graduated from Guy's Hospital in 1977 and after working in general practice in New Zealand, returned to England where he undertook a two-year homeopathic apprenticeship and attended courses run by the Faculty of Homeopathy in London. Charles gained his MFHom in 1982 and since then has been running a busy holistic private practice in Surrey. In the early 1980s he attended the Greek Seminars in London where he was inspired by George Vithoulkas and Vassilis Ghegas. He continues to attend numerous seminars by internationally renowned homeopaths and is particularly excited by the work of Rajan Sankaran, Massimo Mangialavori and Jan Scholten. His other main areas of interest are nutritional and environmental medicine, food intolerance and gut function.

Charles is a founder member of the Oxford Group (HPTG), a founder member of the British Society of Nutritional Medicine in 1984 (now the British Society for Allergy, Environmental and Nutritional Medicine) and also works at Biolab, the UK's foremost nutritional laboratory.

Alice Greene qualified as a doctor in Ireland in 1977. Following a career in general practice in Dublin and London, she gained her membership of the Royal College of General Practitioners. Feeling dissatisfied with drug prescribing as her only option, Alice went on to study classical homoeopathy at the Royal London Homeopathic Hospital, gaining membership of the Faculty of Homeopathy in 1981. She has used homeopathy regularly in practice since. She is a founder member and core teacher of the Oxford Group (HPTG), training doctors, nurses and vets in homeopathy for the last 12 years, and with whom she runs postgraduate supervision groups for doctors. In 2002, she was awarded Fellowship of the Faculty of Homeopathy.

Pursuing her interest in the links between profound relaxation and self-healing, Alice studied autogenic therapy in 1986 and has used it in her work for the last 18 years. Following her chairmanship, she was awarded Fellowship of the British Autogenic Society in 2001 for her services to autogenic training and education.

Alice has also completed a professional training in therapy and counselling with the Psychosynthesis and Education Trust, and sees clients for therapy in addition to her medical work. She holds diplomas in autogenic therapy and psychosynthesis therapy and is a UKCP (United Kingdom Council for Psychotherapists) registered psychotherapist.

For the last 15 years, Alice has established a multidisciplinary holistic medical practice in Harley Street in London, using non-drug approaches to illness and well being.

See www.dralicegreene.com

Peter Gregory graduated from Bristol University in 1972 and worked in mixed practice in his native Sheffield before emigrating to Australia in 1977. After seven years as a partner in a mixed practice in tropical Queensland, he returned to the UK and became interested in homeopathy. He found this to be a logical system of medicine which involved treating animals with understanding and compassion, and using medicines that addressed the underlying disease process rather than simply taking away the symptoms. Peter practised homeopathy both here and in Australia and obtained VetMFHom status in 1991. Shortly afterwards he began to teach homeopathy to fellow professionals. He now works in a holistic veterinary medicine centre in Sussex and continues to teach both in the UK and overseas. He was awarded Fellowship of the Faculty of Homeopathy in 2004.

Peter says that, compared to orthodox practice, working in homeopathic referral allows him to meet clients and patients on a different level, and to gain deep satisfaction from the work; it is this opportunity which he wishes to share.

Brian Kaplan is a classical homeopath and has been a member of the Faculty of Homeopathy since 1983 and a Fellow since 2002. He has been an enthusiastic teacher since the late 1980s and in 1991 was co-founder of the Homeopathic Professionals Teaching Group (HPTG) which continues to teach classical homeopathy to doctors, vets and nurses.

In 1987 Brian co-edited (with Dr Marianne Harling) D.M. Gibson's *Studies of Homoeopathic Remedies* (Beaconsfield Publishers). He has always been deeply interested in the homeopathic method of taking a medical history and in 2001 published *The Homeopathic Conversation* (Natural Medicine Press).

For the past ten years Brian has practised Provocative Therapy, a cutting-edge use of humour and reverse psychology in medicine and psychotherapy. Like homeopathy, Provocative Therapy embraces a contrarian approach. When warmly and humorously encouraged to continue their self-defeating patterns of behaviour, patients quickly choose to prescribe, own and enact their own solutions to their problems.

More information and reviews of *The Homeopathic Conversation* can be seen on Brian's website www.drkaplan.co.uk More information on Provocative Therapy can be found at www.provocativetherapy.co.uk

David Owen has been in full-time homeopathic practice for 20 years, in Winchester, Oxford, Bournemouth and Basingstoke, where he runs busy integrated multidisciplinary practices (www.thenaturalpractice.com). Whilst studying homeopathy in the UK and abroad, David has sought to understand and build on the fundamental assumptions and insights which different teachers have to offer. This has led him to develop his own holistic approach to case analysis and to study Materia Medica from an emotional perspective.

David teaches with enjoyment and inspiration, using a variety of teaching methods to suit different material. Enthusiastic about facilitating groups, he believes a strong learning group such as an HPTG year group can offer enhanced educational opportunities.

David is a founder member of the Oxford Group (HPTG) and has played a key role in developing the HPTG postgraduate supervision programme. For several years he has co-ordinated a module on complementary and alternative medicine for medical students and nurses at Southampton University and is active within the Faculty of Homeopathy, of which he is a past President. David has a vision of homeopathy being practised as a discrete profession but fully integrated with other conventional and complementary approaches to health care; as he describes it: 'returning the heart to medicine'.

John Saxton qualified in 1964. He worked in general mixed practice for five years before moving into purely small animal work. Following his introduction to homoeopathy, this became a steadily increasing part of his work. He attended the training courses at the Faculty of Homeopathy, obtaining his Membership in 1988 and his Fellowship in 1996. He has both taught and examined for the Faculty since 1988, and joined the HPTG in 1995. John now lectures nationally and internationally on their and his own behalf. In 2003 he left general practice and is currently involved with homoeopathic referral work together with teaching and writing.

Robin Shohet is an individual and marital psychotherapist, trainer and management consultant. He is co-author, with Peter Hawkins, of *Supervision in the Helping Professions* (2000, Second edition, Open University Press). He has been teaching supervision through the Centre for Staff Team Development (www.cstd.co.uk) for 25 years. Robin strongly believes that those in the helping professions need to have plenty of space for reflection on their work to avoid burn-out, and is currently writing a book on supporting teachers sponsored by the Teacher Support Network.

Robin lives with his family at the Findhorn Foundation, a spiritual community in the north east of Scotland, and is a member of the Findhorn Foundation consultancy service. In 1999 he organised an international conference there on forgiveness, and intends to run another on the Greek island of Skyros in September 2005. He has been very influenced by The Work of Byron Katie, a revolutionary approach to solving problems (www.thework.org), and its similarity to other non-dualistic teachings. He has taken The Work to India, New Zealand, South Africa and Greece.

The Homeopathic Professionals Teaching Group (HPTG)

The Homeopathic Professionals Teaching Group (HPTG), is a multi-disciplinary training organisation for training health professionals in homeopathy. The trainers are committed to excellence in training and practice.

Originally based in Oxford (UK) and sometimes called the Oxford group, HPTG now teaches in several UK locations and runs international courses. HPTG runs one year part-time foundation courses leading to internationally recognised primary care qualifications in homeopathy, which concentrate on first aid, acute prescribing and basic philosophy. Successful candidates in the examinations can apply to become Licensed Associates of the Faculty of Homeopathy (LFHom). This leads into a part-time course taken over two to three years which prepares participants for examination for full membership of the Faculty of Homeopathy (MFHom).

HPTG runs advanced training and supervision for those working in homeopathy, supporting, educating and developing homeopaths in the personal, practical and organisational issues important to practice. Further information about HPTG and its courses and teachers are available from HPTG, 28 Beaumont Street, Oxford, OX1 2NP or www.hptg.org.